D1338601

THE NUMBER ONE BESTSELLER

JAMIE OLIVER

The Return of the Naked Chef

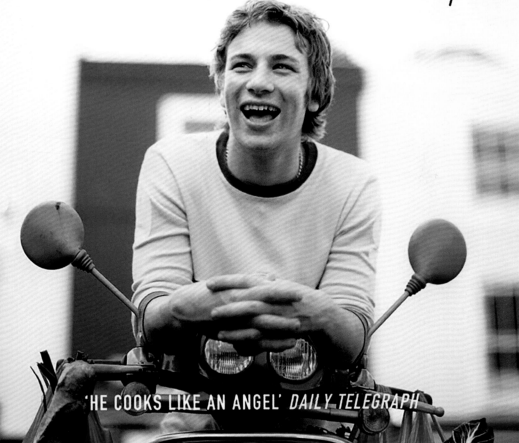

'HE COOKS LIKE AN ANGEL' *DAILY TELEGRAPH*

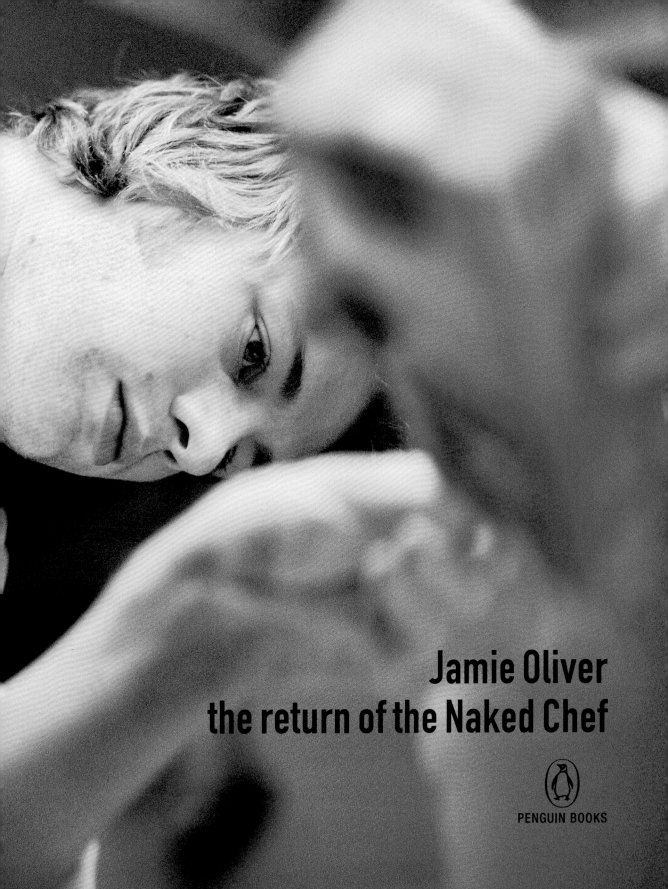

Jamie Oliver
the return of the Naked Chef

PENGUIN BOOKS

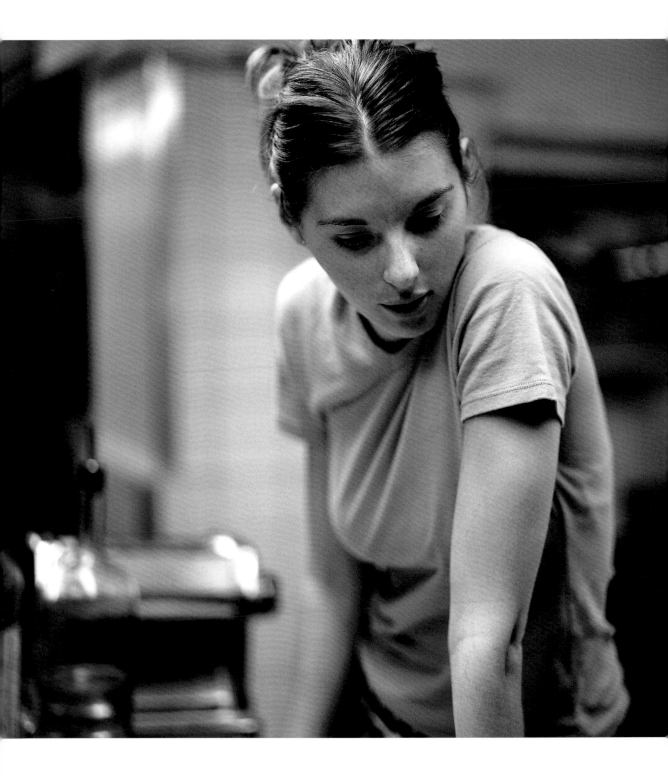

Dedicated to my beautiful missus . . .
The lovely Jools xxx

PENGUIN BOOKS

UK | USA | Canada | Ireland | Australia
India | New Zealand | South Africa

Penguin Books is part of the Penguin Random House group of companies
whose addresses can be found at global.penguinrandomhouse.com

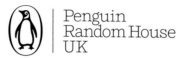

First published by Michael Joseph 2000
Published in Penguin Books 2002
Reissued in this edition 2019
001

Printed in China

A CIP catalogue record for this book is available from the British Library

ISBN: 978–1–405–93352–0

penguin.co.uk

jamieoliver.com

www.greenpenguin.co.uk

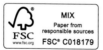

Penguin Random House is committed to a
sustainable future for our business, our readers
and our planet. This book is made from Forest
Stewardship Council® certified paper.

contents

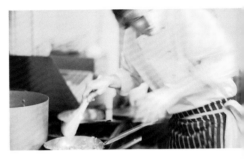

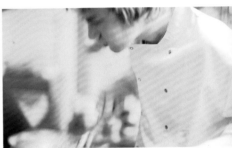

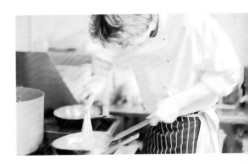

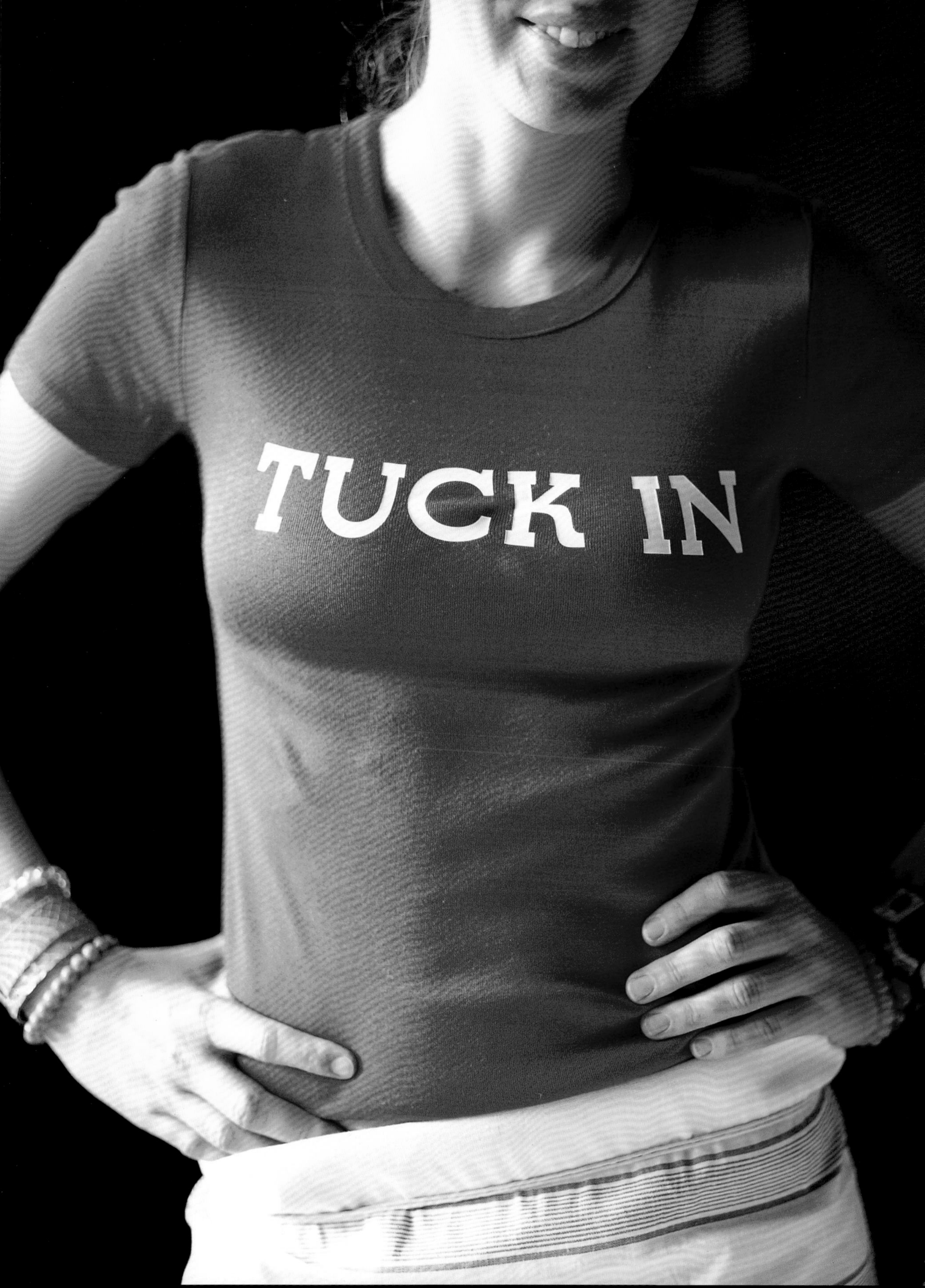
TUCK IN

introduction

Blimey, what a year! If I'd been told a year and a half ago that I would be sitting here now writing my second book as a follow-up to *The Naked Chef* I would never have believed it. Having the chance to write the first was amazing, but to be allowed another crack of the whip is just superb. And am I ready for it? Yes, surrounded by the pukka people at Penguin, good friends and family, you better believe it. I'm gagging for it!

As you can imagine, being the youngest chef on the block, having a bestselling book as well as a cracking television series, not to mention being a bit scruffy and coming from Essex, I've come in for quite a bit of stick from folk. I don't mind. In fact, I quite enjoy it. It makes me laugh. This book isn't about cheffy food, it's for normal people who want shortcuts and tips; people who want to make simple day-to-day meals different and absolutely fantastic or something a little bit more fruity and indulgent. At the end of the day, it's for everyone who is interested in cooking tasty, gutsy, simple, commonsense food and having a right good laugh at the same time. That's what food's all about. It's not just about eating. To me it's about passing the potatoes around the table, ripping up some bread, licking my fingers, getting tipsy and enjoying the company of good friends or family. Pass us the mustard, Dad.

The response to *The Naked Chef* from the media and
thought that I would have been asked to cook at No. 10 for
meeting? What a great buzz that was. Or hearing Zoë Ball
tuna for dinner? Can't get better than that. Or having Mrs
I'm washing my hair. And some of the letters I received
saying they've cooked from the book for the in-laws in dodgy

There was one occasion when I thought I would have to
of the road shouted out, 'Oi, you, Naked! Come 'ere. I want
me, I waited for him to walk over, only for him to say in an
kitchen three nights a week cos my missus says if that
weeks if I'd a seen ya, I'd a knocked your 'ead off.' Then his
it. I think I'm a good chef. So thanks mate, respect.' And I
bill.' And then there were the old ladies in Sheffield – right
said, 'OK love, sign us this book here. Make sure there's
and we love your lingo, don't we, Gwenda?' 'Yes, yes, we do,
you with your clothes on. Can't you get your kit off?' Now I
like a beetroot. I wanted to say something smart back but

I've spoken to loads of strangers while shopping in the
me constructive feedback. This has probably taught me the
massively influenced my approach to this book. Yeah, I still
Naked Chef: using the *bare* essentials of your larder and
But I'm also keen to make use of new ingredients which are
and pulses to fresh herbs and oils from different regions of
quality will definitely improve. PS Check out the index where

the public has been absolutely fantastic. Who would have
Tony Blair and the Italian prime minister at their summit
on the radio say that she'd cooked Fatboy Slim my seared
Merton offer me her baked pasta recipe? Not today love,
were fantastic. It's amazing getting a letter from someone
situations and scored massive brownie points. God bless ya.
leg it, because some bloomin' great geezer over the other side
a word.' Holding on to my vitals, with my life flashing before
aggressive voice, 'Thanks to you mate, I'm in the bleedin'
blond young boy can do it, so can you. For the first couple of
voice softened and he said, 'I really enjoy it now I've got into
said, 'Thanks mate. All the best. I'll send you the laundry
tigers they were. While constantly patting my bottom they
kisses on it. Now, we love your programme, we love your book
Maureen. Pukka, wicked it is. But we're a bit surprised to see
don't get embarrassed easily, but these OAPs had me blushing
every time I opened my mouth I sounded like Scooby-Doo.
supermarkets and walking down the street who have given
most about what real people at home really want and it has
believe in the two things that resulted in my name of the
stripping down restaurant methods to the reality of home.
now being stocked in your average supermarket, from fruits
the world. If we all support these ingredients then variety and
you'll find the V sign pointing out the vegetarian recipes.

make life easy

Before you start cooking, I can't stress enough how much every kitchen should be stocked with the basics. Do this once and get it done properly instead of buying bits and pieces. Buy the ingredients listed here, which I promise won't cost you the earth and will keep you in good stead for the coming year.

S M E G

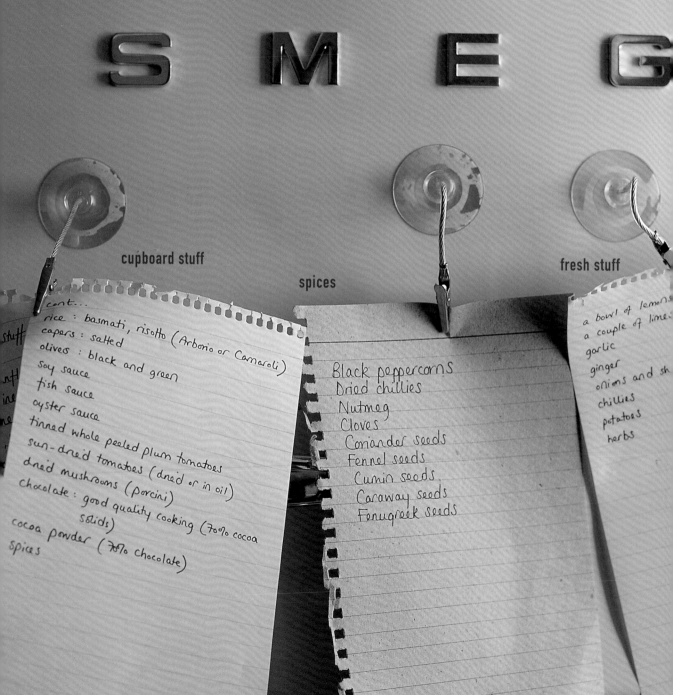

cupboard stuff

spices

fresh stuff

cont...
rice : basmati, risotto (Arborio or Camaroli)
capers : salted
olives : black and green
soy sauce
fish sauce
oyster sauce
tinned whole peeled plum tomatoes
sun-dried tomatoes (dried or in oil)
dried mushrooms (porcini)
chocolate : good quality cooking (70% cocoa solids)
cocoa powder (70% chocolate)
spices

Black peppercorns
Dried chillies
Nutmeg
Cloves
Coriander seeds
Fennel seeds
Cumin seeds
Caraway seeds
Fenugreek seeds

a bowl of lemons
a couple of limes
garlic
ginger
onions and sh
chillies
potatoes
herbs

cupboard stuff

- Oils: extra virgin olive, olive, sunflower, sesame
- Vinegars: red wine, white wine, balsamic, rice wine, herb
- Mustards: Dijon, wholegrain, English
- Maldon sea salt
- Sugar: brown, icing, caster, demerara
- Flour: plain, self-raising, strong pasta (fine strong) Tipo '00', strong bread, corn
- Baking powder
- Dried yeast
- Fine semolina, polenta, couscous
- Dried pasta: spaghetti, linguine, farfalle, pappardelle
- Pulses (dried or tinned): cannellini and flageolet beans, lentils, chickpeas, pearl barley
- Rice: long-grain, risotto rice, such as Arborio or Carnaroli
- Nuts and seeds: walnuts, almonds, hazelnuts, Brazils, cashews, pine nuts, chestnuts, sesame seeds
- Anchovies in olive oil
- Capers: salted (small ones are best)
- Pickled gherkins
- Creamed horseradish
- Low-salt soy sauce, fish sauce
- Tinned whole peeled plum tomatoes, sun-dried tomatoes in oil
- Dried porcini mushrooms
- Quality dark chocolate (70%), cocoa powder
- Runny honey
- Porridge oats, ground bran
- Dried fruits: apricots, raisins, dates
- Light coconut milk

fresh stuff

Obviously fresh stuff is perishable but there are still some basic things that you will always use. I try to have these ingredients available all the time: a bowl of lemons, a couple of limes, garlic, ginger, onions and shallots, chillies, potatoes, herbs.

spices

Spices are a must. They're non-perishable and they're generally as cheap as chips. The fact that an essential spice and flavouring from a certain part of the world can be kept in your kitchen just waiting to be used is fantastic. By lightly roasting and/or pounding, the spices come alive in smell and flavour. There are classic combinations involved in curries, stews and seasonings, but just a single spice with salt and pepper and a little olive oil can turn an ordinary piece of fish or meat into a more classy, subtle and interesting meal. Generally, I prefer to go to small ethnic shops for my spices, as they tend to be better produced, sourced and stored. And they're a hell of a lot cheaper than your supermarkets or delis. Shop for: black peppercorns, dried red chillies, nutmeg, cloves, coriander seeds, fennel seeds, cumin seeds, caraway seeds, fenugreek seeds, cinnamon, cardamom pods, paprika, cayenne pepper, saffron.

potty about herbs

I'm mad about herbs — so much so that I actually have dreams about seeing big patches of them and feeling the utmost pleasure at having them right there at my culinary disposal (how weird). They're an absolute must for any kitchen, whether at home or in a restaurant. I split fresh herbs up into two sections: hardy herbs and delicate herbs. Here's my advice for getting them at their best and cheapest.

fresh herbs

hardy herbs

I'm not a gardener, and I certainly haven't got green fingers, but having grown a selection of rosemary, bay, thymes, sages, marjoram, oregano and mint in window boxes and pots over the last six years, I reckon I've had enough experience to tell you that it's so cheap and dead easy to do. It doesn't matter where you live, or how much space you've got — I've only ever had a garden once (the rest of the time it's been window boxes for me) and even then I found that potted herbs suited me best. Just spending £15 or so on a selection of herbs will give you an exciting range of flavours and you'll have them right there at your disposal — just with a snip of your scissors. So here's how to pot them, bearing in mind that you don't have to pot from seeds:

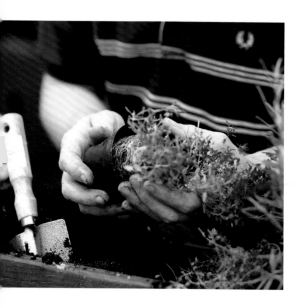

- *From seed*
Scatter your chosen seeds over some good organic soil in a seed tray. Place them somewhere warm and sunny, and keep them watered. When they have sprouted to about 2.5cm high, transfer the seedlings into small pots.

- *Small pot*
Obviously the ideal place to grow your seedlings to the size of the classic market- or shop-bought herb is a greenhouse, but a south-facing window sill will serve just as well. Good soil, good drainage and a small, but consistent, amount of water every other day will ensure a hardy, tasty baby herb, ready to be planted outside.

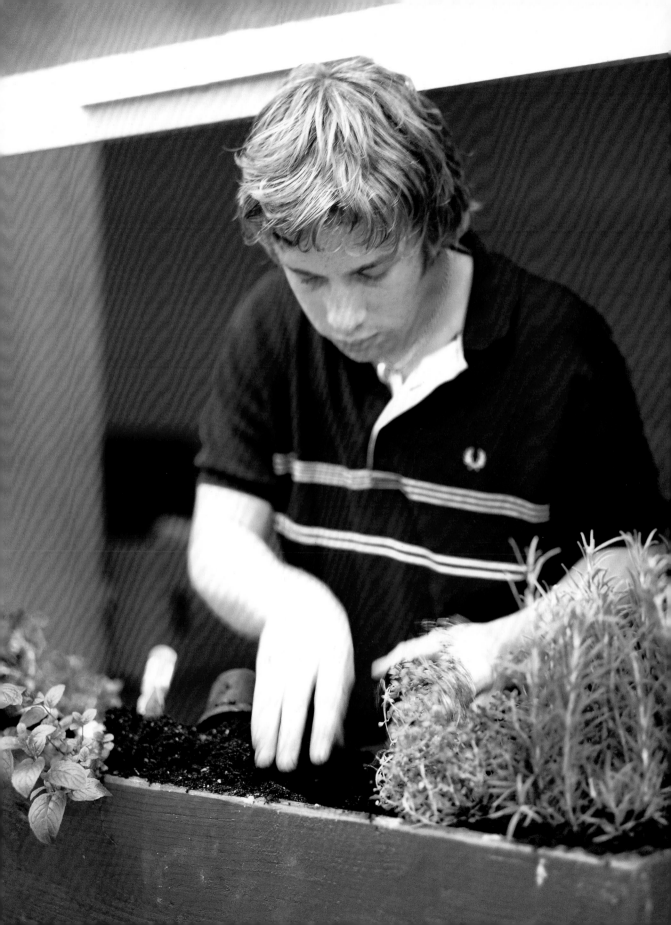

- *Transplanting*

  You can buy herbs ready for planting in the garden or you can use your own baby herbs grown from seed (see page 16). Carefully remove the herb plant from its pot and transplant it into your garden, window box, hanging baskets or large terracotta pots. Make sure you scatter a layer of stones on the bottom of the planting hole, then some good organic soil, before putting the plant on top. This will ensure good drainage. The larger the amount of soil around the herb, the bigger the plant will grow, so bear this in mind.

  When transplanting herbs I tend to use the bigger, more substantial ones like rosemary, bay and sage to shape a bed or pot. The gaps can be filled in with thymes, marjoram and oregano – all are ideal. Mint spreads itself around like mad, and might be better in a pot on its own.

  If you think your herbs need moving to a larger pot or space in your garden at any time, then feel free to do this.

- *Picking & pests*

  Try to pick the new shoots, to encourage the plant into more growth and fullness. Herbs such as oregano and mint tend to die back in cold weather but they grow back with a vengeance in the warmer half of the year. Grow camomile and yarrow near your herbs to keep them healthy, and deter slugs with crushed glass or Vaseline-rubbed pot rims. To get rid of aphids, add a small amount of detergent to some water in a watering can and use this at the first sign of trouble (make sure you wash your herbs thoroughly before using them).

delicate herbs

Quite frankly, I've never had success with growing delicate herbs like flat-leaf parsley, basil, coriander and tarragon. You need a good amount of nutritious soil in a sheltered, light part of the garden, which I've never had (aah), and they will only last for the summer. Lots of my friends have had success using pots inside the kitchen on a bright window sill, but I'm far too impatient so I just buy nice big bunches from the market.

dried herbs

Two scenarios here:

1. The herbs are doing so well they've gone mad and are nicking too much space in the garden or pot, so I have to be brutal and cut back the guilty ones to let the others breathe. I then simply bunch up the bits I've cut back, tie them together and hang them up to dry in a warm place (near a boiler, in an airing cupboard, above an oven or just by some hot pipes). They will take about a week to dry out completely.

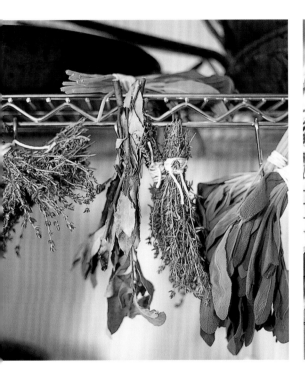 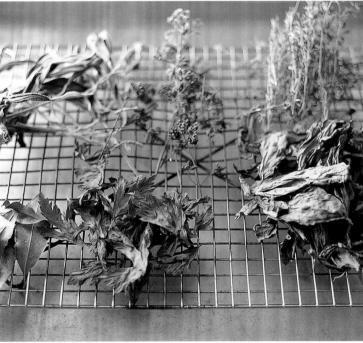

2. I've bought too many herbs from the market or supermarket and I've only used half. I'm not going to be cooking for the next day or two, so I lay them out on a tray and put them in a warm place. Leave them out near the washing machine or something that generates a little bit of heat. Delicate herbs take anything from a day to a week to dry completely and they have so much more flavour and character than your dried sawdusty herbs in packets. Once dried they can be stored in airtight containers for months.

herbs

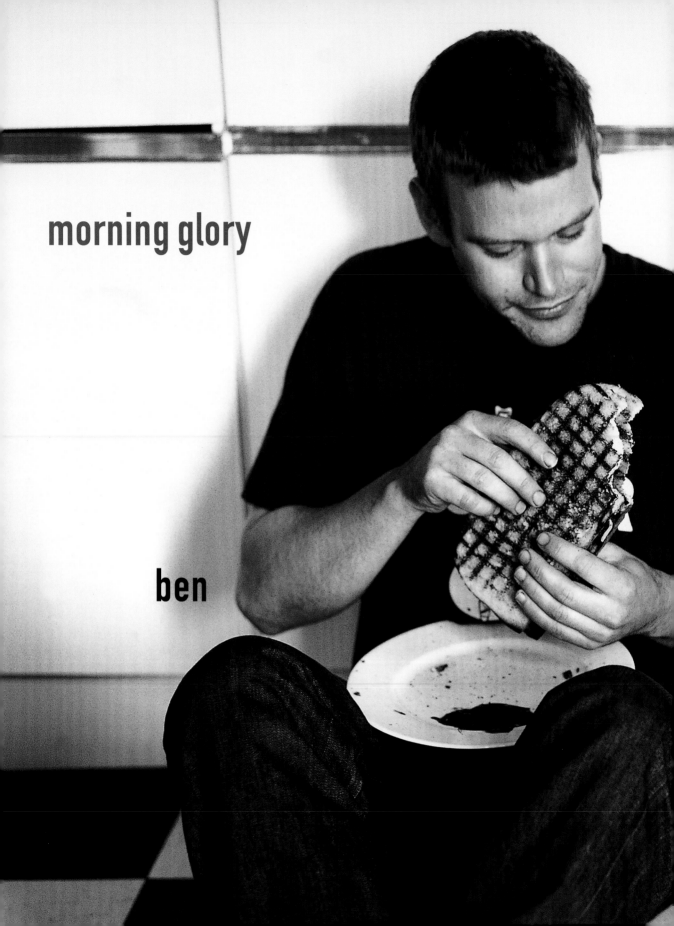

morning glory

ben

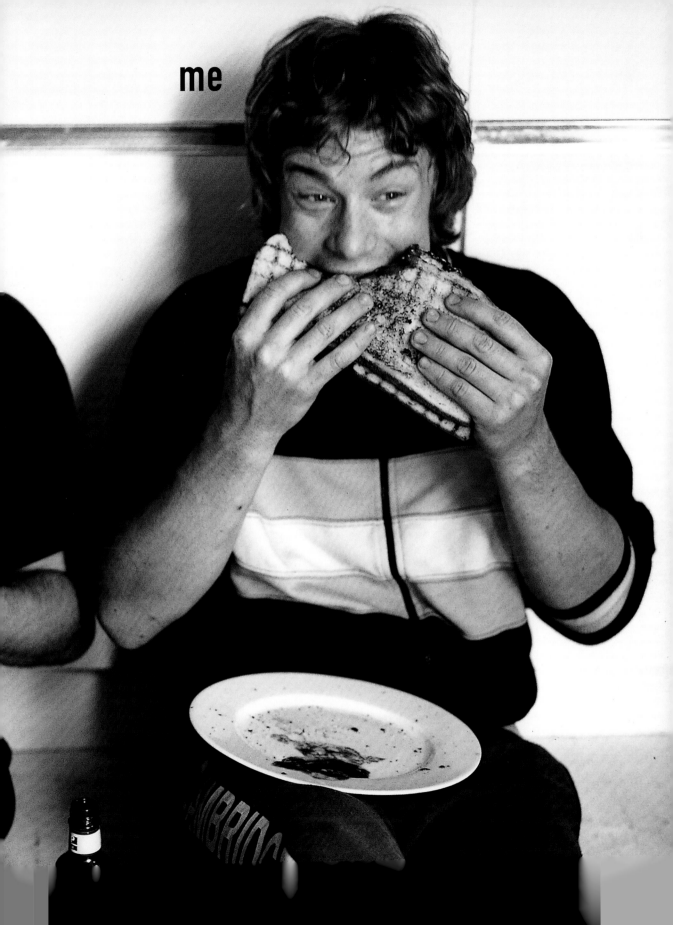

me

I grew up with a mother who cooked us breakfast every single morning, whether it was an unbeatable bacon sarnie, the full monty or her homemade jam and thick-cut bread. She was a star. Now looking back I can really appreciate how well looked after I was, especially when I compare myself to other friends who just got given a couple of Shreddies and some semi-skimmed. 'Breakfast – it's the most important meal of the day,' is what she used to say. My mother was never a worrier but I think she felt a sense of relief if she sent me out the door with a good breakfast inside me because she knew that whatever else happened, I wouldn't starve for the day. She also used to say that your brain needs feeding and that it's at its most effective from seven until eleven in the morning. I'm sure she's right but it didn't do me any good. I still failed miserably at everything apart from art and geology at school, and career-wise I couldn't really see myself as an artistic geologist – all that paint and mud, ooh no.

I think breakfast is one of the most outrageously underrated luxuries in the whole world. Even London as it stands, with its wide variety of restaurants, still offers very little in the way of breakfast. Instead of meetings over lunch or dinner, why not meetings over breakfast? Instead of greasy plastic chairs, why not airy, spacious, fresh and classy diners that serve breakfast from six in the morning until midday? Blooming fantastic, I'd be there. Instead of ingredients bought from the nearest cash and carry, with their classic vacuum-packed bacon and battery eggs, why not a great variety of dry-cured, thick-cut organic bacon and beautiful, golden, free-range eggs from our farmers? After all, there are some that are still doing it properly – it's just a matter of finding them. Fresh juices, self-composed mueslis and homemade breads. I should open up a breakfast diner now before anyone else does – I'd clean up!

The idea of this chapter is not necessarily to make you or your family start eating breakfast every morning. But quite frankly, after a week's work, when the old Saturday and Sunday mornings come along, you don't always have the imagination or the foresight to knock up a quick bit of interesting brekkie for yourself, your family or your partner. If you're after some brownie points and you're a bloke I would highly suggest breakfast in bed for the missus to give you a lucky day, and if you're like my missus, sorry, the lovely Jools, you should attempt a little bit of brekkie for your fella before asking him for a bit of cash for that dress that you've seen in Top Shop. But seriously, before Women's Lib get on the phone, I have so many fantastic memories of breakfast with buddies and I think you'll find some interesting and different things to add to your brekkie repertoire in this chapter. If you know where Pop Tarts originated from then let me know and I'll be over to have some serious words . . . I think it must be in Essex somewhere.

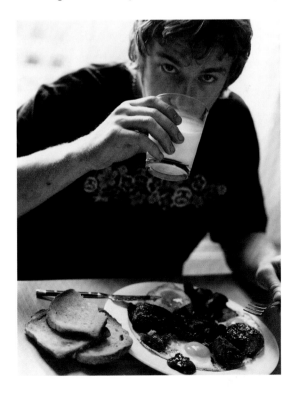

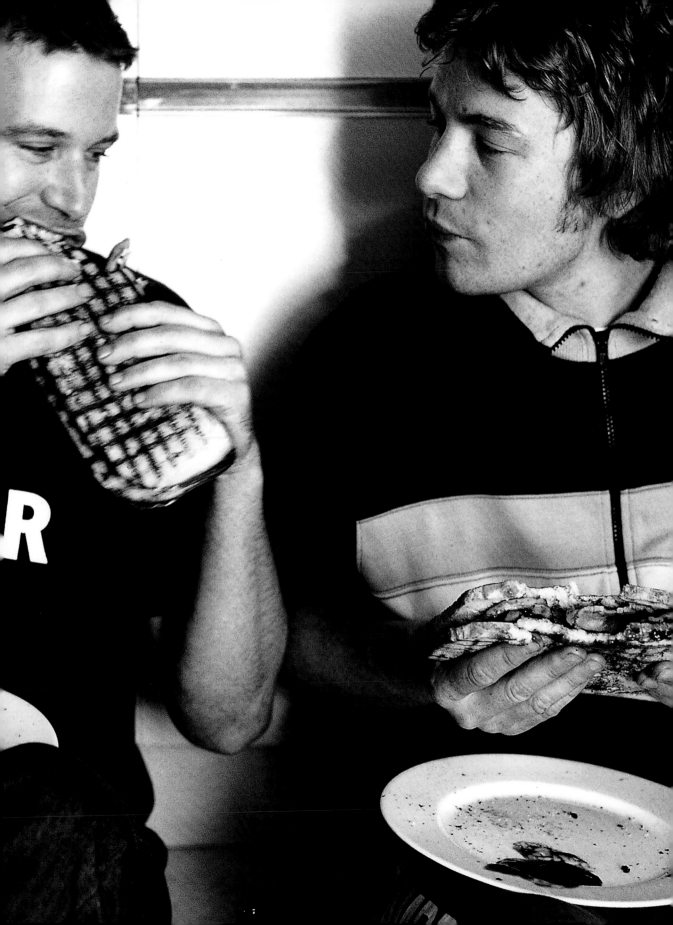

bacon sarnie my stylie

Simple, you may think, but a good bacon sarnie has challenged many chefs, hotels and greasy spoons around the country for years and years. There is a key to this recipe and in my view this is the way to do it.

You need the best dry-cured bacon you can get hold of. This generally means you won't get the shrinkage and watery residue from cooking like you do with most bacon these days. Shame, as we British folk used to be extremely good at rearing and curing good bacon. Second, I would suggest that you try to get hold of thicker-cut bacon; not the wafer-thin stuff that became fashionable a few years ago – you need something you can really get your teeth into. Third, I buy a small, fresh sandwich loaf (gotta be white unless you need your roughage), which should be around 25cm long. I then cunningly and politely ask the baker to slice it lengthways, instead of across as normal. I do this all the time and it's great. It's purely a visual thing but it seems to make it taste better to me – I don't know why. I've always been a strange boy.

So, you've got your bacon and your bread. You could quite easily go ahead and cook your bacon and toast your bread under the grill. Lovely. But if you fancy yourself as a bit of a tiger then acquire a ridged griddle pan, which I get as hot as possible (about 4 minutes on the highest heat) and then begin to grill about 4 slices of bacon (per person if you're greedy like me). After about 1 minute you can turn the bacon over and it will be golden with those funky charred marks across which I also think benefit the flavour slightly. Cook the other side for 1 more minute. At this point I shuffle all the bacon up one end of the pan to carry on cooking a little longer while I toast off my 2 long pieces of bread in the pan. What I love about this way of doing it is that the bread soaks up just a little (not a lot) of the fat that has cooked out of the bacon which makes it even more tasty. When it has toasted on both sides you could butter your toast – I don't bother – and lay your bacon across each slice. Squeeze the 2 bits of bread together. Now it's ready to be eaten, preferably with some HP sauce. In the past I have also added tomatoes and mushrooms to the pan, which do go down very well in the sarnie too.

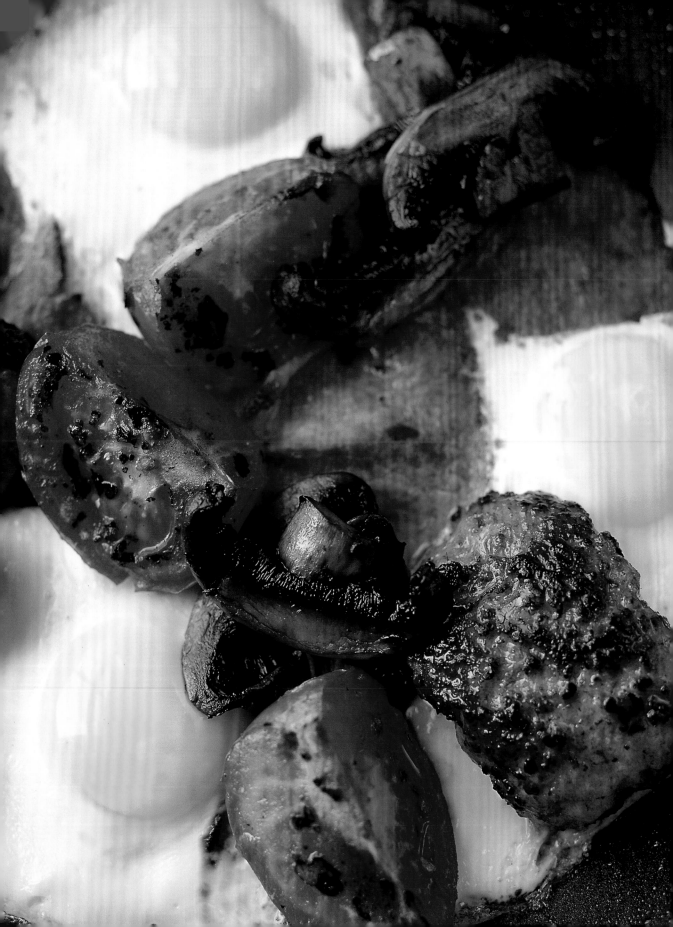

midnight pan-cooked breakfast

Me and this dish go back a long way. To the pre-shaving days of being an under-age drinker down the Wagon and Horses in Saffron Walden with a fake ID and all my village mates. Only once in a while of course. But seriously, without trying to sound like a lagered-up geezer, I think everyone's experienced the need for food around midnight, whether the binge was small or large, otherwise why would kebab shops be so popular in Britain? Anyway, I always used to have three or four friends back to my house for munchies or to stay the night and this dish was devised so we didn't have too much trouble making it or too much washing up to do. In actual fact, I only had to wipe the non-stick pan clean. It also makes its way from the pan to the plate quite quickly, as patience isn't a virtue at that time of night with my mates!

First of all get the biggest non-stick pan available, and preheat it on a high heat while you gather your ingredients. Obviously you wouldn't be organized at this point so it's a matter of using what you've got, but ideally I like to have mushrooms, bacon, tomatoes, sausages and eggs. By the time you have got these together the pan will be hot, so slice your sausages in half lengthways and pat them out flat so they cook quickly. Place in the pan at one side. On the other side, put a tiny lug of oil and place a pile of mushrooms over it which you can rip up or leave whole. Shake the pan about a bit to coat the mushrooms and season with some sea salt and black pepper. Push to one side, then lay some slices of bacon and halved tomatoes in the pan. Cook for a couple more minutes until the bacon is crisp and golden. Shake the pan and turn the bacon over. Now is the time to put a round of toast into the toaster.

At this stage you should respect the rustic and authentic look and shuffle everything about so that it's all mixed together and add 2 or 3 eggs at different ends of the pan. The whites of the eggs will dribble in and around the sausages, bacon, tomatoes and mushrooms. Turn the heat down a little and continue to cook for another minute before placing the pan under the grill and finishing the eggs to your liking. Using a non-stick pan I've always found the removal of this dish to the plate extremely easy – it will resemble a frisbee and will slide on to your plate with no trouble at all. Doesn't that sound appetizing? But honestly, it really is a gem.

figs, honey & ricotta

I first had this in Florence for brekkie and my initial reaction, as the unworldly person that I am, was why am I having cheese for breakfast? But this combination of perfect figs and honey is amazing, different and damn tasty.

Before you say you don't like figs … that's what I used to say, remembering chewing on tough, tasteless old figs that you would have to peel the skin off. But I have been converted because the shops and supermarkets are starting to get hold of really good fresh figs, both green and purple. Slightly firm on the outside, soft and sometimes sticky in the middle, with an amazing sweet taste – unlike anything else.

There's no point in me giving you amounts for this recipe as, quite frankly, you can have as much or as little as you like. Myself, I normally go along the 1 fig per person vibe. Score a criss-cross across the top of the fig to about halfway down, then gently squeeze the base of the fig. It will pucker up and look extremely funky, and helps us by exposing a little of the inside which we can drizzle honey in. Place the fig beside a slice of fresh ricotta from the deli counter at the supermarket. Drizzle the fig and the cheese generously with your favourite honey and tuck in. I have been known to squash both the ricotta and the fig with a fork on to some buttered toast – tuck into that as well, it's all good stuff.

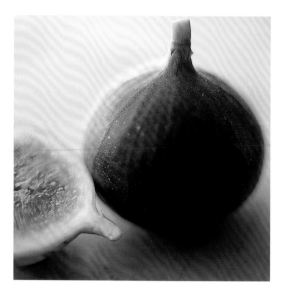

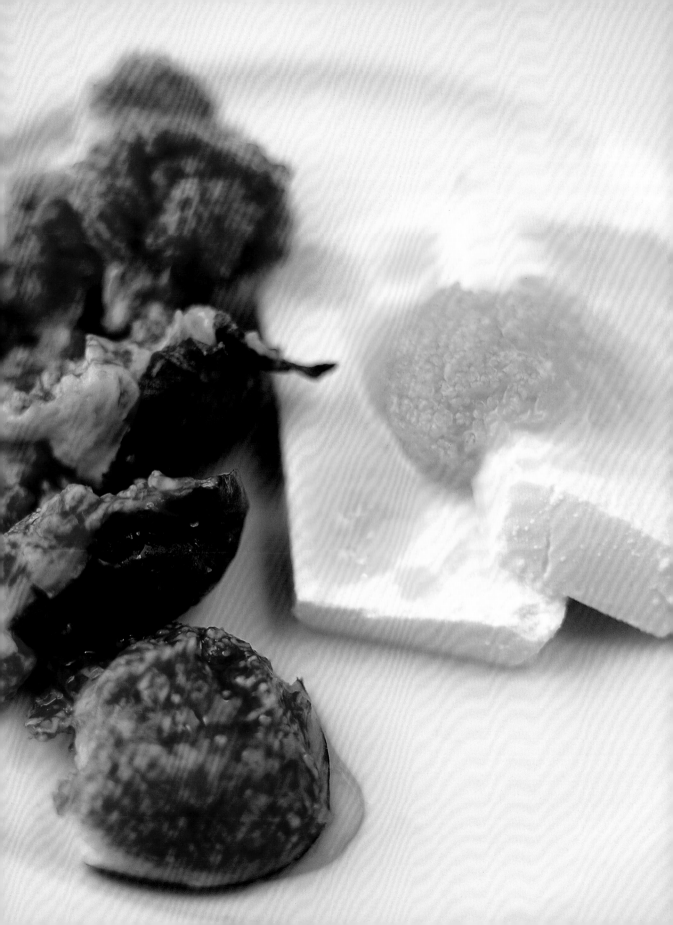

beef tomatoes, basil, ham & mild cheese on thick toast

This is something my dad used to make me on holidays in Cyprus from the hotel's self-service breakfast bar. I've finally found a purpose for the good old beef tomato – for this recipe they are fantastic.

This brekkie or snack takes precisely 1 minute to make. So in go 2 slices of thick breawd to the toaster. While toasting, you need to slice your tomatoes as thick as you like, get out a couple of small sprigs of basil, some sliced ham, which I like to remove the fat from, and some mild cheese. Out comes your hot toast. Place it on a plate and very lightly rub it with a garlic clove sliced in half (it's a gesture and it's breakfast, so don't go OTT but it's well worth doing). Drizzle with some good olive oil – you could butter it if you fancy but I think oil keeps in with the Mediterranean thing. Simply place on the tomatoes – very important, season now with sea salt and black pepper. Rip over the basil. Lay on the ham and cheese and tuck in. Very simple, very tasty.

PS A nice poached egg on top does the trick if you've got the extra time.

CALORIES	FAT	SAT FAT	PROTEIN	CARBS	SUGAR	SALT	FIBRE
412kcal	17.4g	5.8g	17.2g	49.9g	5.5g	3.2g	3.7g

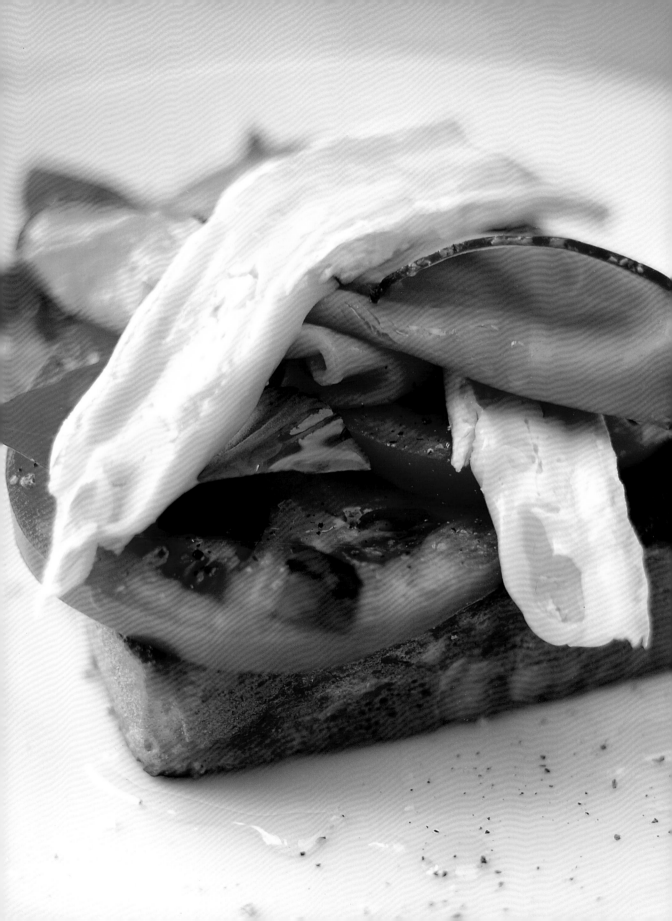

pukkolla

Pukkolla is my name for this outrageously scrumptious concoction. It's one of the best things you can have for breakfast as it's got everything you need to kickstart your day. Basically it's a bastardized, personally composed muesli. The great thing about it is that you can adjust it to your own preference. It's very handy to have a large plastic airtight container to store your composed pukkolla in, so try and get hold of one.

composing & preserving

serves 12
8 large handfuls of organic Scottish porridge oats
2 large handfuls of ground bran
1 handful of chopped dried apricots
1 handful of chopped dried dates
1 handful of crumbled walnuts
1 handful of smashed or chopped almonds, hazelnuts or Brazil nuts

Put the porridge oats and bran into your plastic container with the apricots and dates. Add the walnuts and your other chosen nuts (I usually bash them up in a tea towel). At this point feel free to improvise, adding any other preferred dried fruits like raisins, sultanas or figs – but personally I think my combination works pretty well. This will keep for a good couple of months very happily in your airtight container, but you'll have eaten it by then, I guarantee.

making & knocking together

milk, to cover
½ a crunchy apple per person

I would definitely try to make this the night or day before you want to eat it, although it can be made at the time (but you won't get the smooth silky scrumptious texture that the milk gives it overnight). I normally place double the amount of composed cereal I need (i.e. 4 portions for 2 people) in a bowl. Doubling up like this gives you enough to eat for the next couple of days. Cover with milk, grate in around ½ an apple per person and stir immediately to stop the apple discolouring. Place in the fridge.

tucking in & eating

½ a banana per person
runny honey, to taste

Remove the bowl from the fridge. You will find that it has softened and thickened, so loosen with a little milk. Add your banana, sliced or squashed. You will find that a lot of natural sweetness has come out of the dried fruit, so add honey to taste. Serve in a bowl with a dollop of yoghurt and some mixed berries, if you like.

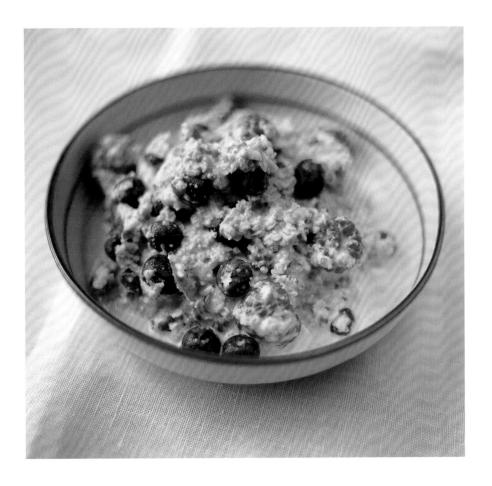

CALORIES	FAT	SAT FAT	PROTEIN	CARBS	SUGAR	SALT	FIBRE
227kcal	5.7g	1.9g	9g	37.7g	21.9g	0.2g	5.1g

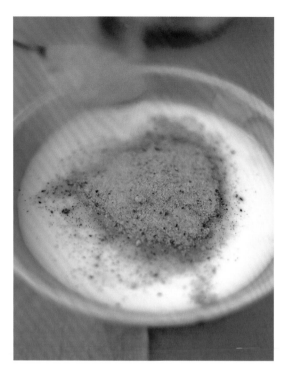

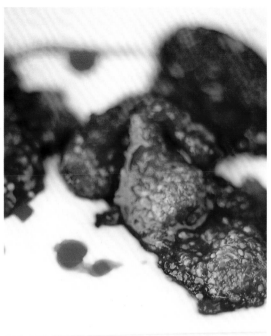

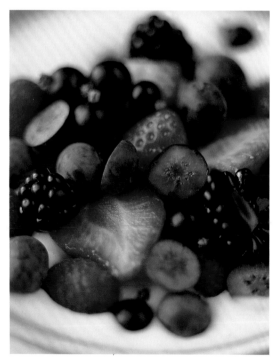

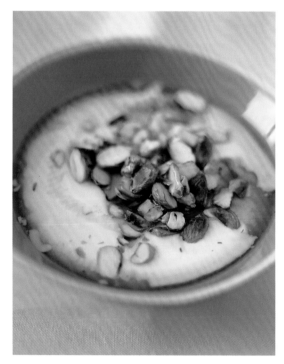

homemade yoghurt

I love making yoghurt. For some reason it's really rewarding, I'm not sure why. I think it's the fact that it's so damn easy to turn a litre of milk into a litre of yoghurt. Things like yoghurt and bread are fantastic for kids to make, so let them have a go.

1 litre full cream milk
1 × 500g tub of live yoghurt

Bring the milk to the boil in a thick-bottomed pan, then turn the heat off. Leave for around 40 minutes, or until the milk has cooled down to body temperature. Use your finger to check. At this point stir or whisk in your live yoghurt. Cover and leave at room temperature for 6 to 8 hours, by which time you'll be amazed to see that the milk has turned into creamy yoghurt. Without getting too technical, the live culture in the yoghurt turns the natural sugar of the milk into acid. This causes the milk to thicken and taste slightly sharp. Different yoghurts may react slightly differently, i.e. some will thicken more than others, but, as a rule, all results are fantastic. Place it in the fridge to chill. It will keep for around a week.

Here are some of my favourite ways to eat yoghurt for breakfast or dessert, but don't forget it's great in marinades (see page 194) and fantastically refreshing lobbed over spicy lamb and couscous or curry and rice:

- With vanilla sugar
- With strawberries marinated in balsamic vinegar (see page 256)
- With mixed soft fruit
- With rosewater, honey and pistachio nuts
- With pukkolla (see page 32)
- With figs and a bit of brandy
- With baked fruit

CALORIES	FAT	SAT FAT	PROTEIN	CARBS	SUGAR	SALT	FIBRE
71kcal	4g	2.6g	3.7g	5.2g	5.2g	0.1g	0g

THESE VALUES ARE BASED ON 100G

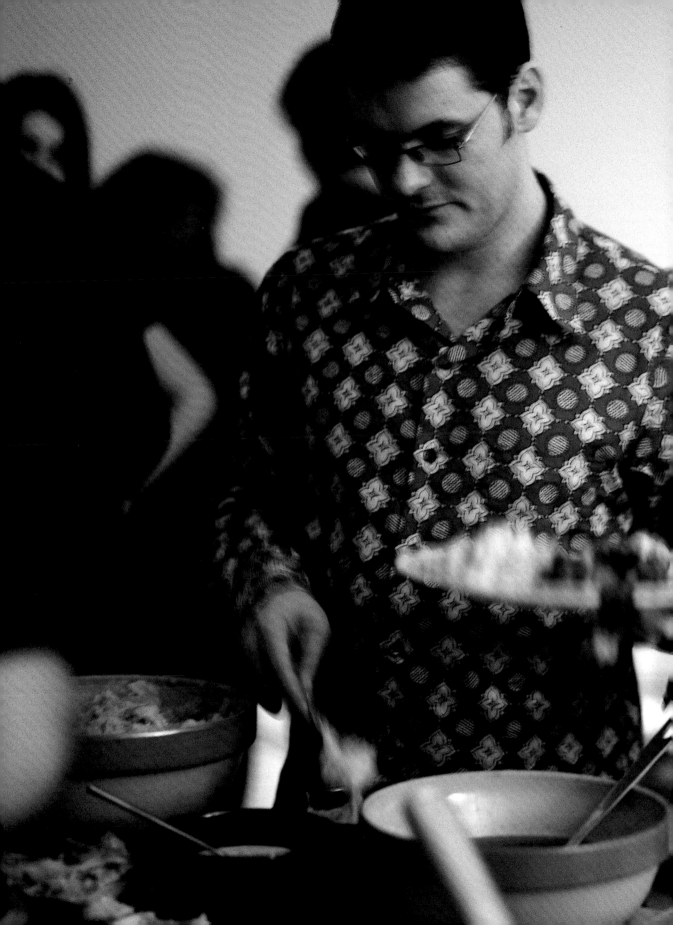

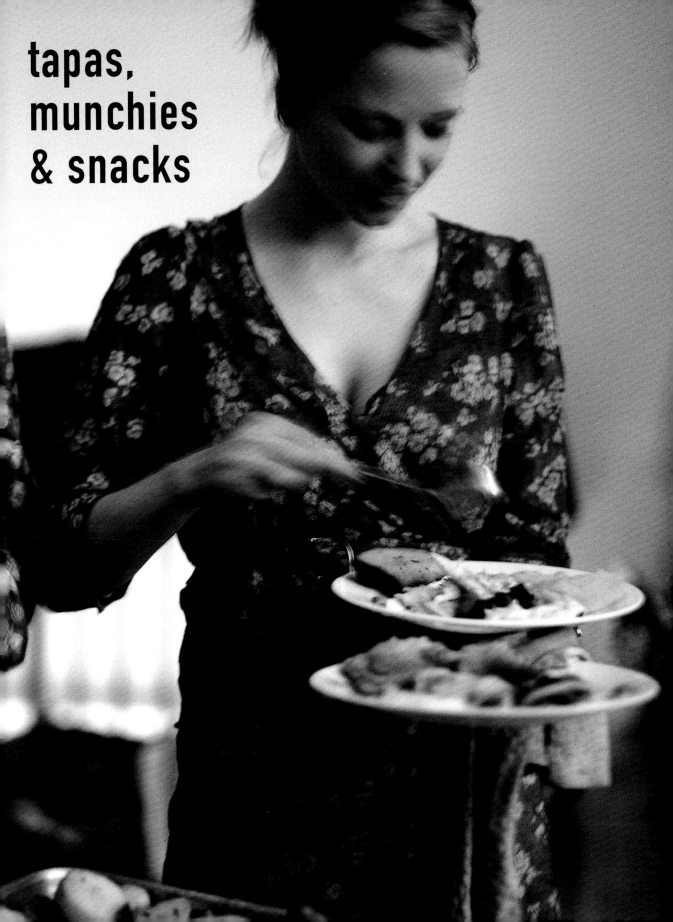

tapas,
munchies
& snacks

I'm a right one for munchies and snacks, and the whole tapas thing really gets me going. I must admit I love the old Boxing Day dinner so much that I do constantly try and re-enact it for the rest of the year with the snacks in this chapter. My missus, sorry, the lovely Jools, often finds me watching telly late at night after work or a band practice gnawing on some stale old bread, pickled chillies and various other preserved or recycled dinners. She always looks disgusted by my new and innovative combinations but sod it, I'm happy.

When having friends over for drinks, or if people just pop round, it's fantastic to offer them a little nibble of something. If you've got a couple of simple tricks up your sleeve they'll think you're a right little tiger and that you've made a bit of an effort for them. If you're a bit of a midnight muncher like me then check out this chapter for some finger-, bite- and snack-sized tucker.

Any combination of dishes in this chapter works extremely well but personally I like to serve them with some interesting homemade bread. Try my flatbreads (see pages 235–6) as they will go brilliantly with everything in this chapter.

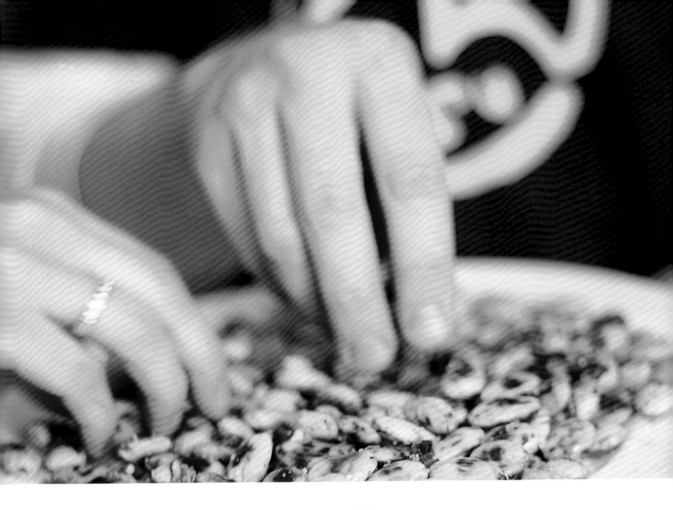

pan-toasted almonds with a touch of chilli & sea salt

These must be the quickest thing in the world to make. Believe me, there's nothing more scrumptious with any cold drink and good company than a plate of hot, toasted, tasty almonds. Try throwing them into salads too – nothing better.

serves 8
½ tablespoon olive oil
250g blanched almonds
1–3 small dried red chillies

Put the oil and almonds into a hot frying pan. Fry and kinda toast the almonds until golden brown, shaking the pan regularly to colour them evenly and accentuate their nutty flavour. Crumble in the chilli to taste and add 2 generous pinches of sea salt. Toss over and serve hot on a large plate. Bloomin' gorgeous.

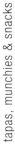
tapas, munchies & snacks

CALORIES	FAT	SAT FAT	PROTEIN	CARBS	SUGAR	SALT	FIBRE
200kcal	18.3g	1.5g	6.6g	2.2g	1.4g	0.5g	2.3g

smashed spiced chickpeas

This is a bastardized humous recipe, but no less tasty. I love it best spread over thin pizza bases (see page 232) cooked on a hot griddle pan until charred, but tortillas are always a quick option.

serves 6
1 × 400g tin of chickpeas, drained, or use 170g dried ones,
   soaked and cooked until tender
1 good pinch of cumin seeds, pounded
1–2 small dried red chillies, crumbled
1 clove of garlic, peeled and pounded
1 lemon
extra virgin olive oil

This is so simple to make. Really it's all about personal taste – the way I look at it is that chickpeas are really moreish but they need a good kick up the backside to really get their flavours happening. So by smashing them up and adding a good pinch of cumin for a bit of spice, a little dried chilli for a touch of heat, garlic for a bit of ooorrrggghhh, a good squeeze of lemon juice to give it a twang and seasoning to taste with sea salt and black pepper, you pretty much hit the nail on the head. Then add oil to loosen and flavour. Love it.

CALORIES	FAT	SAT FAT	PROTEIN	CARBS	SUGAR	SALT	FIBRE
86kcal	4.9g	0.7g	3.5g	7.6g	0.5g	0.3g	1.8g

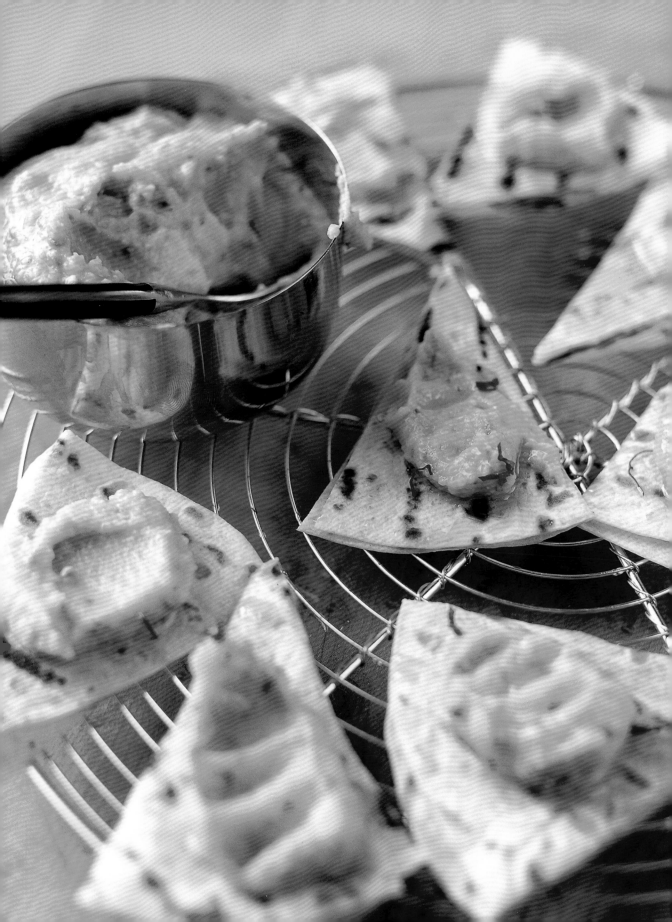

black olive tapenade

Olives with stones in are much tastier – they will make all the difference to this tapenade.

serves 6–8
250g black olives, stone in
1 clove of garlic, peeled
6 anchovy fillets, in oil
extra virgin olive oil
1 lemon

Destone the olives by squeezing or bashing them and removing the stone. You can either very finely chop the olives, garlic and anchovies by hand or place them in a food processor and whiz until smooth. Taste and season with sea salt and black pepper, add oil to loosen and, very importantly, squeeze over lemon juice to taste.

CALORIES	FAT	SAT FAT	PROTEIN	CARBS	SUGAR	SALT	FIBRE
77kcal	7.9g	1.2g	1.1g	0.2g	0.1g	1.6g	0g

blackened sweet aubergine

Some people call this 'poor man's caviar' but I say it's 'Essex boy's caviar'.

serves 6–8
4 firm aubergines
1 pinch of cumin seeds, pounded
1 clove of garlic, peeled and pounded
extra virgin olive oil
2–3 lemons
optional: 1 handful of fresh coriander, basil or flat-leaf parsley, chopped

Preheat the oven to full whack (240°C/475°F/gas 9). Place the aubergines on a tray and cook for 1 hour, or until the insides are very soft. Remove from the oven, slit the skin and scrape out the insides. Add your cumin and garlic, stir in and break up. You can make this smooth or coarse, depending on how you feel. Add oil to loosen. Squeeze in the lemon juice and season to taste. I would never serve this hot, but it's great just warm or at room temperature. If adding herbs do this at the last minute, roughly or finely chopped.

CALORIES	FAT	SAT FAT	PROTEIN	CARBS	SUGAR	SALT	FIBRE
75kcal	5.1g	0.8g	2.5g	5.8g	5.2g	0g	0.1g

tapas, munchies & snacks

smashed courgette paste

This is fantastic spread over toast, thrown into pasta or even in ravioli with ricotta. Try to buy small firm courgettes as they have a better flavour and are not all soft and fluffy in the middle.

serves 6–8
olive oil
2 cloves of garlic, peeled and finely chopped
1–2 small dried red chillies, crumbled
6–8 small courgettes, unevenly sliced
1 good handful of fresh mint, leaves picked and chopped
1 lemon
extra virgin olive oil

Put a couple of lugs of olive oil into a hot pan and fry the garlic and chillies for a couple of minutes. Throw in the courgettes, stir around and coat. Turn the heat down slightly and put the lid on. Give the pan a shake and stir every 5 minutes for around 35 minutes, making sure the courgettes don't catch on the bottom. Cooking with the lid on will help stop it drying out. When the courgettes are really soft, with some chunky pieces and the rest almost pulped, remove from the heat and taste carefully. Remembering that this will probably be used on bread, you may have to adjust the chilli to taste. Season well with sea salt and black pepper and pour in 4 good lugs of extra virgin olive oil to flavour and loosen. Finally add the chopped mint and squeeze in the lemon juice.

tapas, munchies & snacks

CALORIES	FAT	SAT FAT	PROTEIN	CARBS	SUGAR	SALT	FIBRE
103kcal	9.5g	1.4g	1.5g	3.7g	2.6g	0.4g	1g

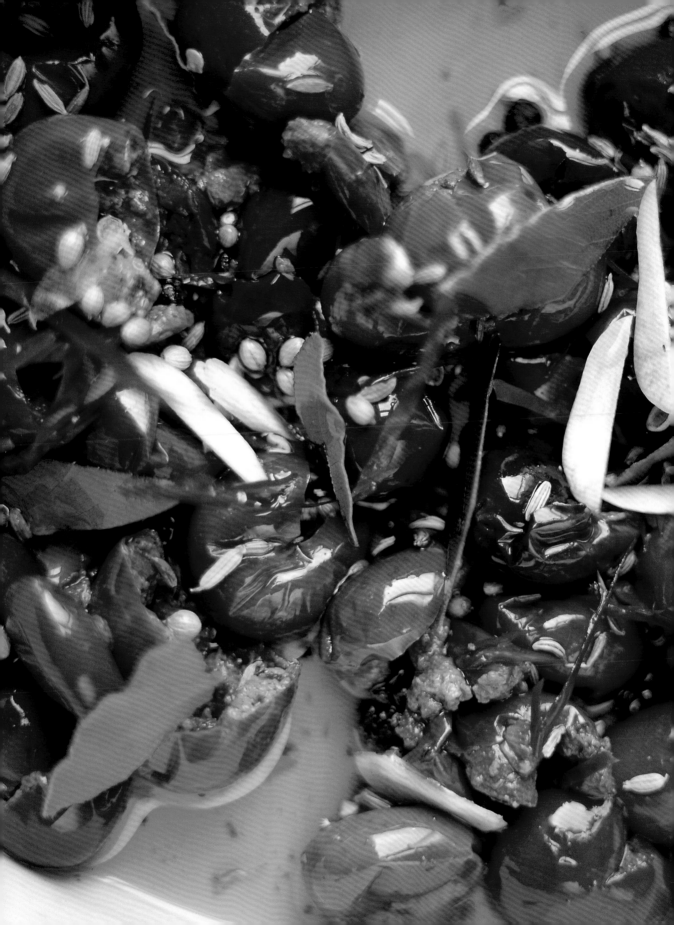

marinated olives

The thing about olives is that there are so many varieties, so when at deli counters in supermarkets, feel free to ask to try all of them. When I've found a type I like, I buy around 500g each time. The olives can then be flavoured with fantastic things – but use dried flavourings if you want the olives to keep well.

Mix your olives in a bowl with a good sprinkling of dried oregano, a ripped-up bay leaf and some crumbled dried red chillies. Season with just black pepper as olives are salty already, and add some cracked coriander seeds or fennel seeds. Then pack the olives tightly into an airtight jar and cover with a good olive oil. This is a fantastic marinade which will complement the olives, making them dead tasty and great for cooking with, using in salads or simply as finger food with drinks.

blackened marinated peppers

Fantastic as part of a tapas or antipasti selection, or serve simply with a piece of grilled fish or in salads.

serves 6
4 large peppers, ideally 2 red, 2 yellow
1 large clove of garlic, peeled and finely sliced
1–2 small dried red chillies, crumbled
1 tablespoon coriander seeds
5 good lugs of extra virgin olive oil
1 splash of red wine vinegar
1 good handful of fresh basil

Normally I place the peppers directly on the naked flame of my gas hob. If you don't have gas, then blacken under the grill or on a barbecue. Once blackened all over, allow to steam in a covered bowl for 5 minutes. Peel and deseed. Don't wash the skins off under running water as you will lose a little of the fantastic sweetness that you've created by blackening them. I normally tear each pepper into around 8 strips and place them in a bowl. Add the garlic, chillies, coriander seeds and oil to the peppers with the red wine vinegar. The key is to season well to taste. Toss this and, ideally, allow to sit for an hour, tossing occasionally, before ripping in your basil and serving.

CALORIES	FAT	SAT FAT	PROTEIN	CARBS	SUGAR	SALT	FIBRE
163kcal	15.6g	2.2g	1.1g	5.1g	4.6g	0g	2.8g

slow-cooked & stuffed baby bell chilli peppers

These are the most fantastic thing. You eat the chillies whole and they are amazing as munchies with drinks, not too hot. At the same time they make lovely flavoured olive oil which I like to add garlic and bay to for extra flavour. Great used on salads, over mozzarella and other cheeses, on pizzas and over pasta.

makes 10 portions
1kg small, round baby bell chilli peppers
1 bottle of olive oil (don't panic – see below!)
1 good handful of fresh parsley or basil, leaves picked
2 good handfuls of rocket
1 small handful of baby capers, soaked and drained
1 handful of anchovies, in oil
10 tablespoons balsamic vinegar, or enough to cover

Halve your chillies, remove the seeds and wash in cold water, then drain. Tightly pack into a large earthenware dish and cover with the oil, then place in the oven at 170°C/325°F/gas 3 for 35 to 45 minutes, or until just tender. Carefully remove the dish from the oven and leave to cool. Take the chillies out of the dish. Pour the fantastic flavoured olive oil back into the bottle it came from. Finely chop the parsley or basil, rocket and capers. Roughly chop the anchovies and mix everything up in a bowl. Just before you want to serve them, dress with the balsamic vinegar, and season. Stuff this filling into the chillies and serve on a plate as tapas.

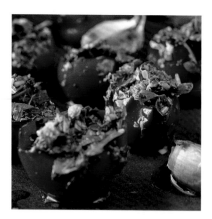

CALORIES	FAT	SAT FAT	PROTEIN	CARBS	SUGAR	SALT	FIBRE
99kcal	5.5g	0.8g	2.1g	10.1g	9.8g	0.7g	2.3g

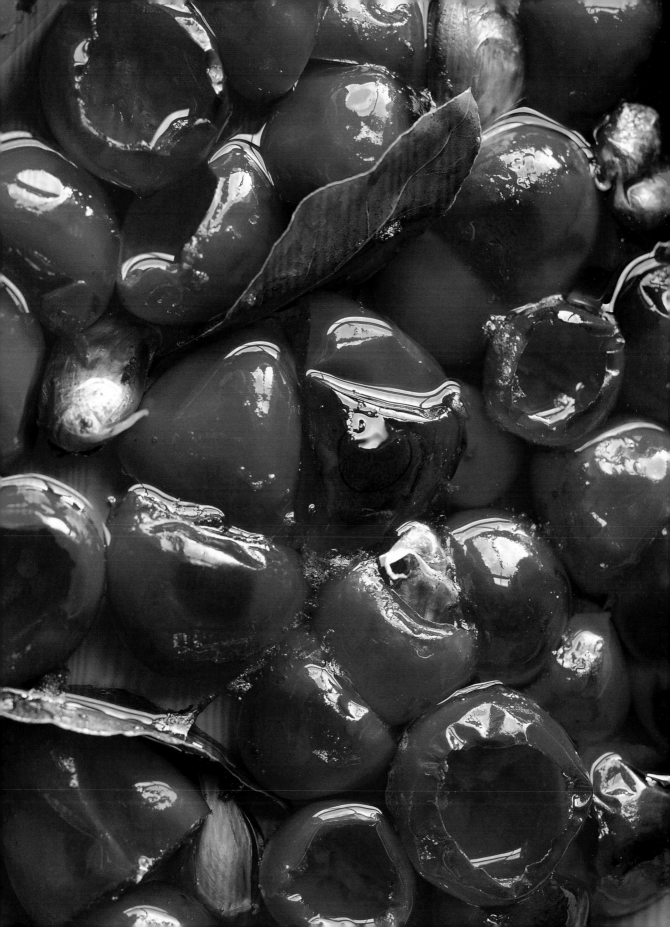

marinated anchovies

Unless you're lucky enough to get fresh ones, the best anchovies you can get hold of are nearly always salted and whole. These are still great for cooking, but to eat an anchovy like you do when you're abroad, draped over toasted crostini, with milky cheeses and in salads, I personally feel no matter how good the anchovy is, the salt overpowers the natural flavour of the dish. So what I do is marinate anchovies to remove their excess salt, then infuse them with other interesting flavours.

Simply take the anchovies off the bone and leave them under running water for a couple of minutes. Pat dry and place a layer snugly in a dish. The main thing is to have something acidic to remove the salt, and a good sweet wine, lemon juice or herb vinegar will do this — add just enough to nearly cover the anchovies. Add the same amount of extra virgin olive oil, then any flavours that take your fancy, such as chilli, fennel seeds, fresh parsley, fresh thyme or flecks of garlic and lemon peel. To make all the difference, marinate in the fridge for between 2 and 16 hours before eating.

grilled butterflied sardines

serves 6–8
1 lemon, peeled
1 small handful of fresh breadcrumbs
1 pinch of dried oregano
1–2 small dried red chillies, crumbled
1 small handful of fresh flat-leaf parsley, leaves picked and chopped
8 large fresh sardines, scaled and gutted

Finely chop the lemon peel, then mix everything, apart from the sardines, together in a bowl and season with sea salt and black pepper. Remove the heads from the sardines and open the belly of each fish. With your left hand pinch away the flesh from the spine; with your right hand pull the spine away from the flesh. It's a bit fiddly, but well worth doing. You will end up with the boned fillets butterflied open. Then all you have to do is press your flavoured breadcrumb mixture on each side of the sardines.

I like to cook the fish on a very hot griddle pan or barbecue. Some of the breadcrumb mix will fall off during cooking but that doesn't matter because it will have imparted its flavour by then and done its job. It literally takes 1 to 2 minutes to cook until crisp. Serve on a plate with a squeeze of lemon juice. Fantastic. Wicked with a glass of wine.

CALORIES	FAT	SAT FAT	PROTEIN	CARBS	SUGAR	SALT	FIBRE
169kcal	9.1g	2.6g	20.2g	2g	0.1g	0.3g	0.2g

marinated squid with chickpeas & chilli

serves 6–8

6 medium squid, gutted and cleaned

1 × 400g tin of chickpeas, drained, or use 170g dried ones,
    soaked and cooked until tender

5cm piece of fresh ginger, peeled and finely sliced

4 lugs of extra virgin olive oil

2 fresh red chillies, deseeded and finely sliced

1 handful of fresh flat-leaf parsley, leaves picked and finely chopped

1 handful of fresh coriander, leaves torn

2 lemons

You can ask your fishmonger to clean the squid for you. Score the squid in a casual criss-cross fashion. This will allow your marinade to get right in there. In a hot griddle or frying pan, or over the barbecue, sear and char the squid. It should take about a minute for the white flesh and a little longer for the tentacles. Remove and slice up the white flesh of each squid into 3 or 4 pieces, leaving the tentacles whole. Put the rest of the ingredients, except the herbs, into a bowl with the lemon juice, season with sea salt and black pepper, then add your squid while still hot and toss everything together. Just before serving, throw in your herbs and check again for seasoning.

CALORIES	FAT	SAT FAT	PROTEIN	CARBS	SUGAR	SALT	FIBRE
187kcal	8.7g	1.4g	19g	8.9g	0.9g	0.3g	0.1g

salted & spiced prawns

serves 6–8

1kg small raw shell-on prawns

6 generous pinches of mixed spices, such as fennel, coriander,
    cumin, chilli, lightly crushed

Leave the shells on the prawns, although you can remove the heads if you want. Get a wok or large pan very hot, then add 4 generous pinches of sea salt and the spices. Toast and toss around for 30 seconds before adding the prawns. Shake vigorously and toss – the salt and spices will stick to the prawns. After a minute or two the prawns will have cooked and changed colour and should be tasty and crunchy. I normally eat the prawn shells but you don't have to.

CALORIES	FAT	SAT FAT	PROTEIN	CARBS	SUGAR	SALT	FIBRE
62kcal	0.8g	0.2g	14.6g	0g	0g	3.9g	0g

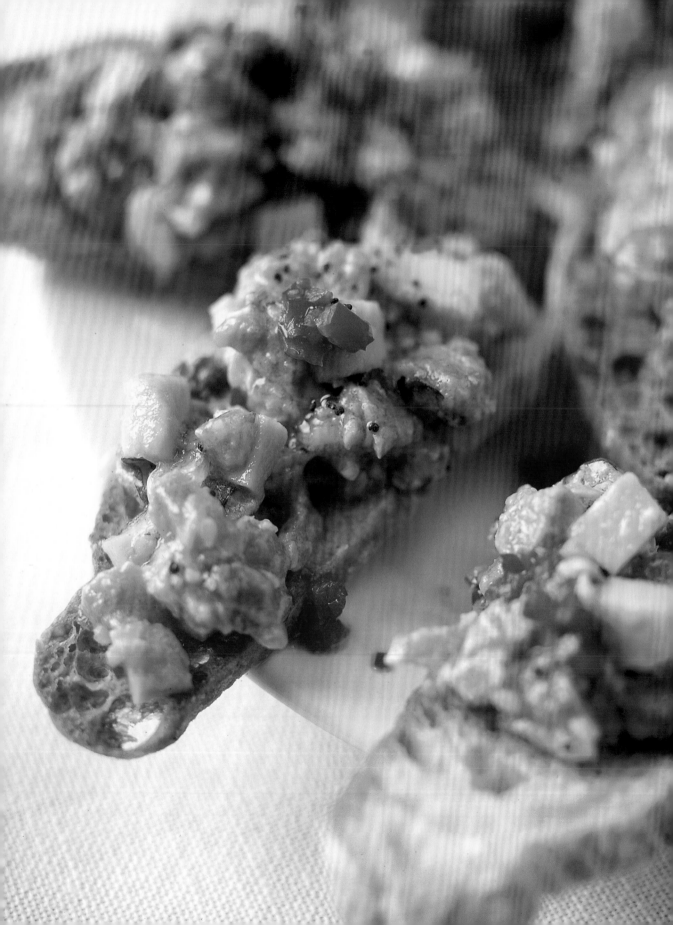

Asian infused tuna

Try to buy firm, deep red tuna. The idea is for it to be eaten raw – just like sushi – but, in actual fact, the acidity of the lime juice starts to cook the fish.

serves 6–8
450g tuna
4–5 limes
1 ripe avocado, peeled and diced
1–2 fresh chillies, deseeded and finely chopped
3 tablespoons sesame seed oil
4 tablespoons coconut milk
1 good handful of fresh coriander, leaves picked and finely chopped
2 heaped tablespoons sesame seeds
2cm piece of fresh ginger, peeled and finely chopped
low-salt soy sauce, to taste

Finely dice the tuna and place in a bowl. Squeeze over the lime juice, then add the rest of the ingredients, adding a little soy sauce to season, if needed. This fantastically flavoured tuna is great on thinly sliced toasted bread.

CALORIES	FAT	SAT FAT	PROTEIN	CARBS	SUGAR	SALT	FIBRE
206kcal	13.2g	2.3g	20.4g	1.4g	1g	0.2g	0.4g

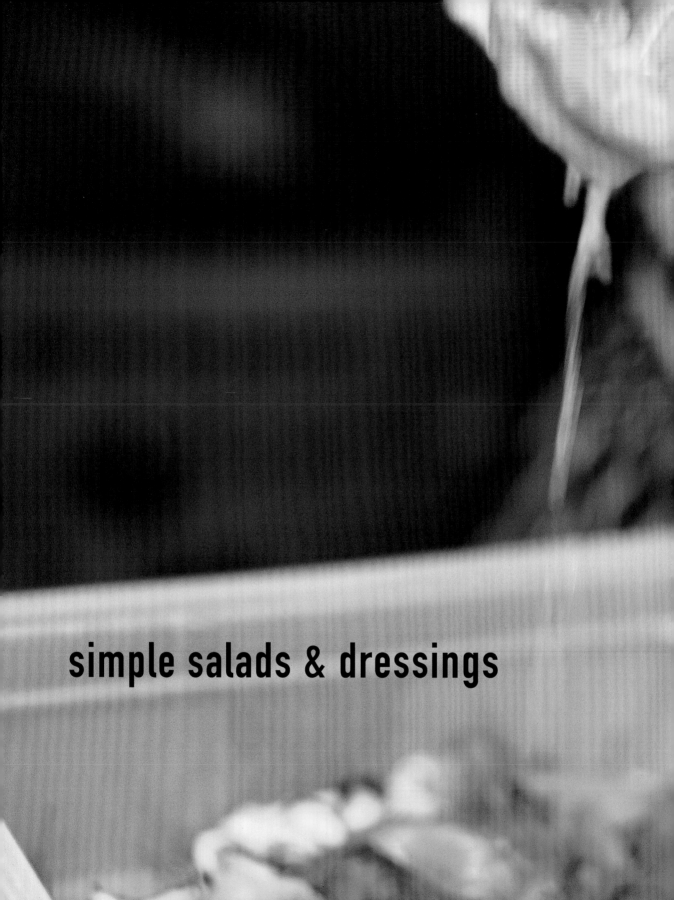

simple salads & dressings

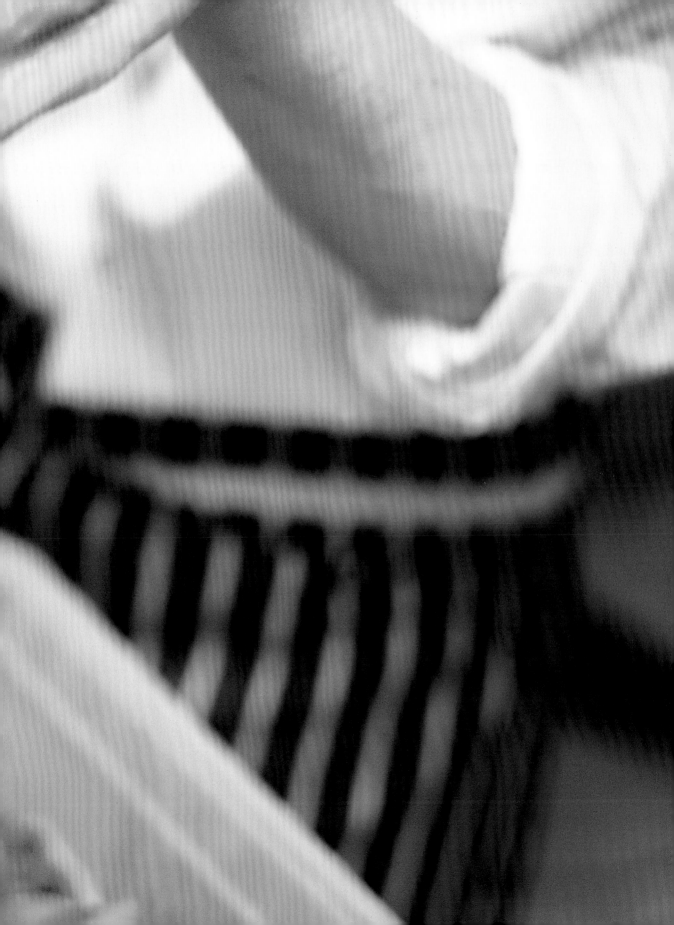

I love salads and, like in the last book, I've made them really simple and conversational. Try to eat salads regularly and you'll really get into them. I've spoken to so many people about what they like to eat, and you won't be surprised that most blokes when asked what they like say 'MEAT', 'MEAT AND TWO VEG' – that means chips and mash. Well, that's great – me too. But you can't beat a good salad. Even when I'm taken out to some of the most expensive restaurants in London I still always ask for the chef's mixed salad even if it's not on the menu. I think it tells you a lot about a kitchen when you order a salad – you will either get one that has been chucked together without much thought or you will get a mixture of fantastic different leaves and herbs which, when eaten, makes you think, 'God, that's nice. What was that I just ate?' A great salad can also simply be one or two things that complement each other. It doesn't have to be complicated.

So to get friendly with salads you should buy a couple of nice big salad bowls that you can put in the middle of the table, acquire some good extra virgin olive oil, some different vinegars – there's so much choice now – and buy some things that you have never thought of trying before. There's loads of new salad leaves, different types of radishes and tomatoes, etc. It's endless. Get stuck in.

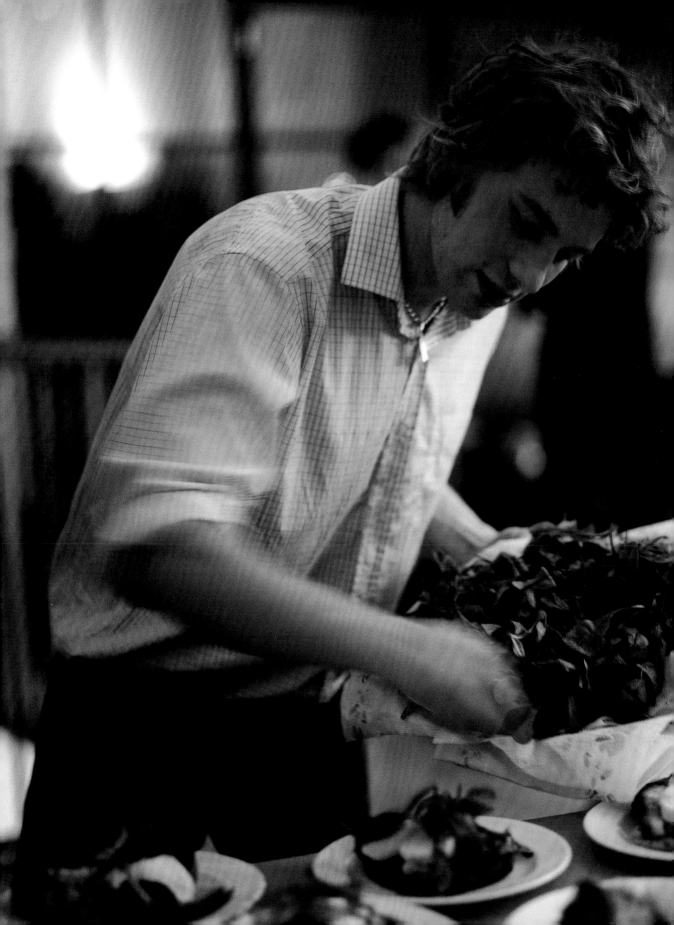

mozzarella & grilled chilli salad

This is a great salad that can get away with being part of an antipasti selection as well as a main course salad or sandwich filling. Simple flavours again: it's all based around the milky soft mozzarella and the slightly more refined heat of the grilled chilli. If possible try to buy buffalo mozzarella, as it's made out of buffalo milk which makes the cheese far more tasty and delicate in both texture and taste. The salad doesn't work nearly as well with that chewy horrible stuff that is used on pizzas.

I normally use 1 fresh red chilli to every ball of mozzarella, but do use more or less as you please. Prick the chillies with a knife, otherwise they can puff up and explode in your face, and place them straight on to the naked flame of a gas hob. If you don't have gas, put them into a pan on the highest setting of your electric hob or under the grill. Either way you need to blacken the chillies on all sides, so turn when need be. When fully blackened, place in a sandwich bag, wrap in clingfilm or cover in a bowl for 5 minutes until cool. This will steam the skins and make peeling and deseeding easier.

While the chillies are steaming, gently rip up the mozzarella into 4 or 5 pieces and randomly place on a large plate. Peel and deseed the chillies and slice lengthways as thinly as you like. It's quite important to scatter them evenly over the mozzarella and very important to wash your hands after doing so before you rub your eyes or anything else! Now rip up some purple and green basil over the top, and sprinkle with sea salt and black pepper. Add a little squeeze of lemon juice and a generous lug of olive oil. Nice one.

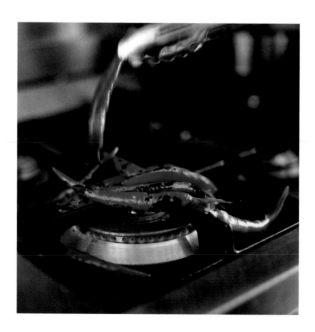

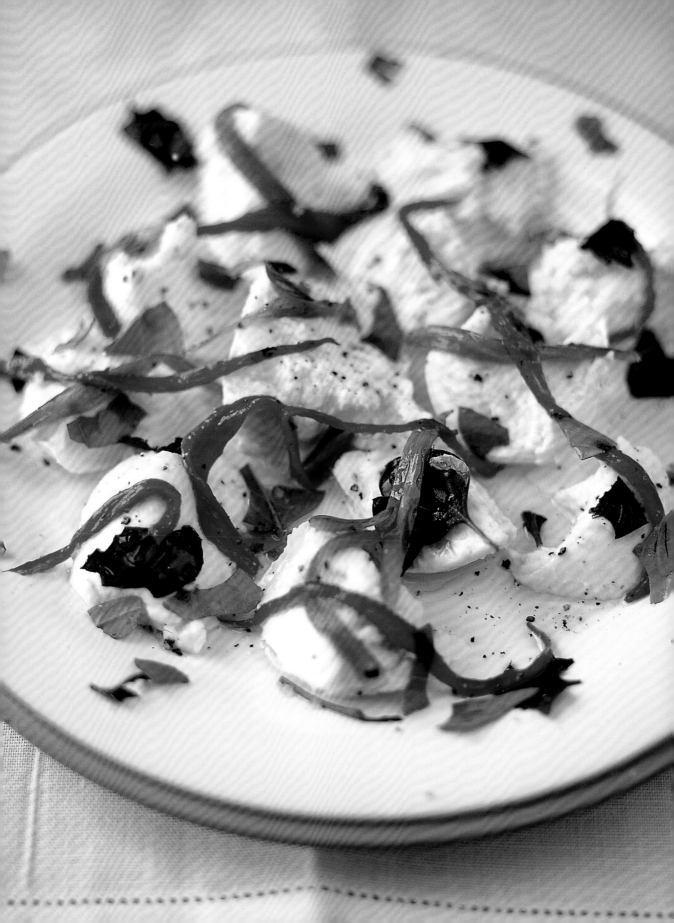

squashed cherry tomato & smashed olive salad

This is probably the quickest salad I make, but no less tasty for that. Very few ingredients, simple flavours, complete sense. Try to make use of the wider range of cherry tomatoes available now: yellow, tiger and plum for instance. And, trust me, it's much better, tastewise, to buy olives with their stones still in than without.

 Always going along the line of 4 parts tomatoes to 1 part olives, simply squash the tomatoes into a bowl. I always have to put one hand over the tomatoes as I do this as juice and pips go everywhere – generally on me. You can be as rough with the tomatoes as you like, as the salad looks much better rough and rustic than perfect and pretty. Then gently smash the olives on a board with a hard object – a cup or a rolling pin. Remove the stones, throw the olives in with the tomatoes and toss together.

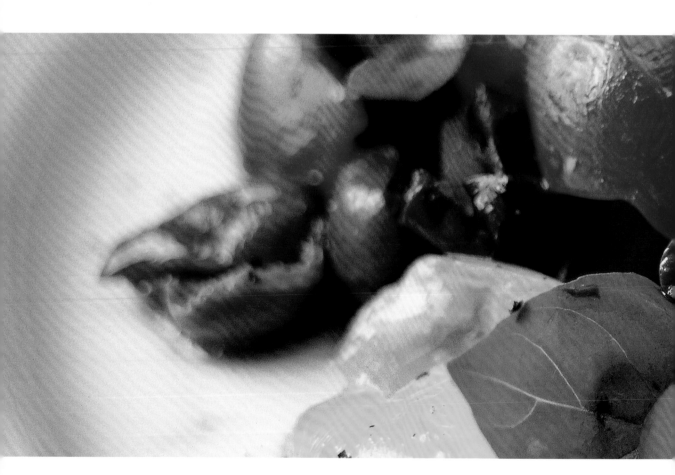

That's the basis of the salad made now, but what you've done already makes complete sense in cooking. Tomatoes need salt, olives are preserved in salt, you've squeezed the juice out of the tomatoes which in return draws the salt and the smoky flavour out of the olives. This makes the olives very edible and the tomatoes damn tasty. That's the most important bit done; all we can do now is enhance it. This can be done to your personal taste with a couple of drizzles of vinegar, preferably red wine or herb, some black pepper and 2 or 3 good lugs of extra virgin olive oil. And just before serving, rip in as much basil as you can afford and even a handful of rocket if you have some. Lovely.

PS If you have any leftovers, toss them in with some hot spaghetti.

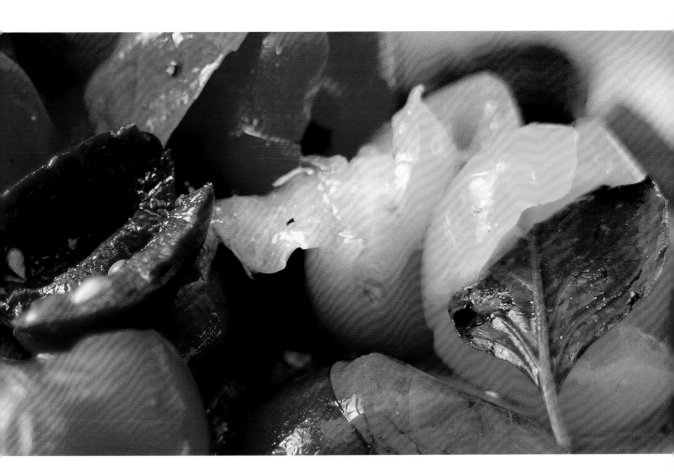

couscous with grilled summer vegetables & loadsa herbs

This couscous recipe is quite a bit different from the norm because instead of boiling or steaming the couscous you just feed it from raw with a really tasty dressing. This means it keeps a slight bite which I think is more interesting for a salad.

serves 4

250g couscous

3 red peppers

1 handful of asparagus, trimmed and peeled, if needed

2–3 small firm courgettes or patty pans, sliced

1 small bunch of spring onions, trimmed and finely sliced

2–4 fresh red chillies, deseeded and finely sliced

3 good handfuls of mixed fresh herbs, such as basil, coriander,
  mint, flat-leaf parsley

2 × olive oil & lemon juice dressing (see page 81)

red wine vinegar

Place the couscous in a bowl with 300ml of cold water. This will start to soften the couscous and you will see the water disappear as it soaks in. While the couscous is softening, we need to blacken the peppers. I do this by placing the peppers directly on to the naked flame of my gas hob. If you don't have gas, then blacken them under the grill or on a barbecue. Once blackened all over, place in a covered bowl for 5 minutes. This will steam the skins and make peeling and deseeding easier. Remove the skins and seeds and roughly chop.

On a very hot griddle pan, lightly char the asparagus and courgettes or patty pans on both sides, then toss them into the bowl of couscous with the peppers, spring onions, chillies and ripped-up herbs. Mix well. Add the extra virgin olive oil & lemon juice dressing and toss well. Finally, taste and season with sea salt and black pepper and a couple of drizzles of red wine vinegar for a slight twang. It's a beautiful thing.

CALORIES	FAT	SAT FAT	PROTEIN	CARBS	SUGAR	SALT	FIBRE
563kcal	32.2g	4.7g	12.7g	59.2g	10.4g	0g	5.1g

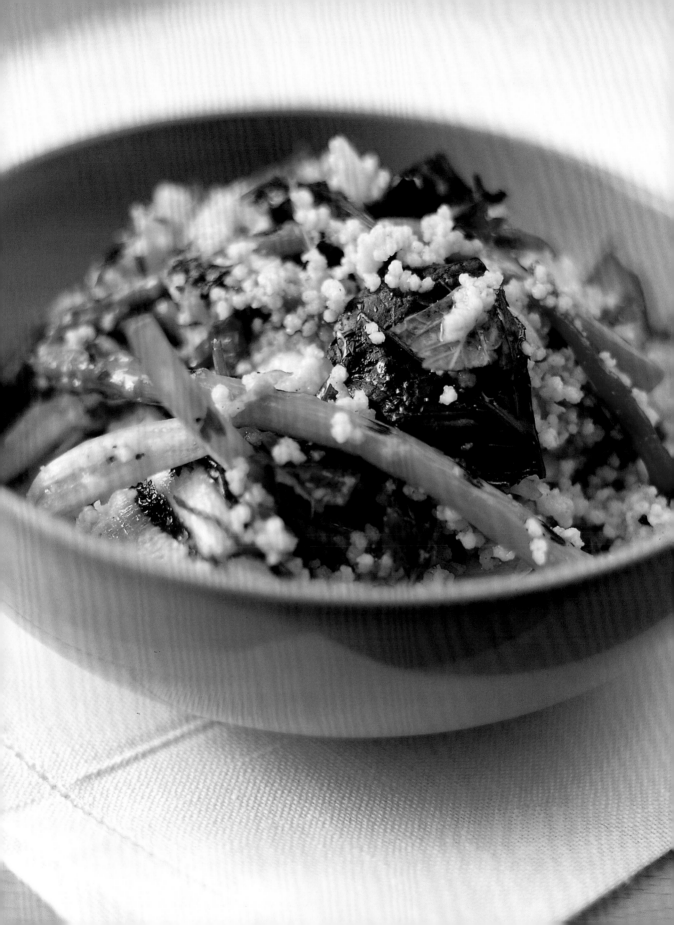

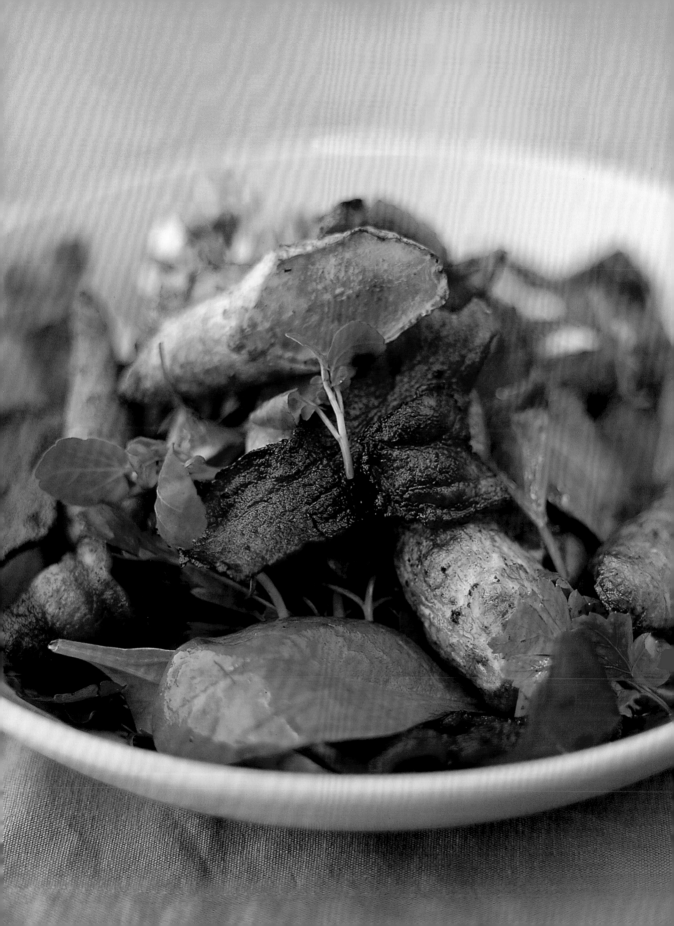

warm salad of winter leaves, bacon & Jerusalem artichokes

As far as salads go, this is a real hearty one, full of flavour and pretty damn gutsy. The idea behind warm salads is that you have interesting and slightly more robust salad leaves, usually mixed with sautéd vegetables or roasted meat. Anything from chicken livers, smoky bacon and scallops to roasted tomatoes, pine nuts and caramelized onions. Smoky bacon and Jerusalem artichokes is a brilliant combination.

Jerusalem artichokes are becoming more common in supermarkets now, but don't confuse them with globe artichokes, which look like big fat thistles. Jerusalem artichokes look more like new potatoes gone mad. For this recipe I normally use around 2 artichokes and 2 strips of bacon per person, but it really is up to you. I also use any combination of radicchio, cos, oak leaf, curly endive, rocket and baby spinach.

Rip the leaves up and place in a salad bowl or on a plate. I prefer to scrub the Jerusalem artichokes instead of peeling them, before cooking in boiling salted water until just soft. Cool under cold running water, drain, and slice as you would sautéd potatoes. Then in a large frying pan fry some dry-cured streaky bacon, which should be sliced across as thick as you like. When golden and crisp, remove from the pan and put to one side. Add the sliced artichokes to the pan with a splash of oil, a little unsalted butter and some sea salt and black pepper. Shake the pan occasionally, putting the bacon back in when the artichokes are golden and crisp. Sprinkle over the salad leaves and drizzle generously with either the basil, balsamic vinegar & pine nut dressing (see page 80) or the mustard & herb vinegar dressing (see page 81).

CALORIES	FAT	SAT FAT	PROTEIN	CARBS	SUGAR	SALT	FIBRE
304kcal	24.3g	8g	6.5g	17.9g	4.3g	1.6g	5.6g

watercress, rocket, sweet pear, walnut & Parmesan salad

What a pukka combination, simple and classy. Don't try to make this when you feel like it, make it when you can buy perfect pears otherwise it will taste naff. For one person I normally use around half a pear, 2 big handfuls of watercress and 2 big handfuls of rocket. If the pear skins are nice I just give them a wash, if not I remove them with a speed-peeler. Cut them in half and deseed. It doesn't really matter

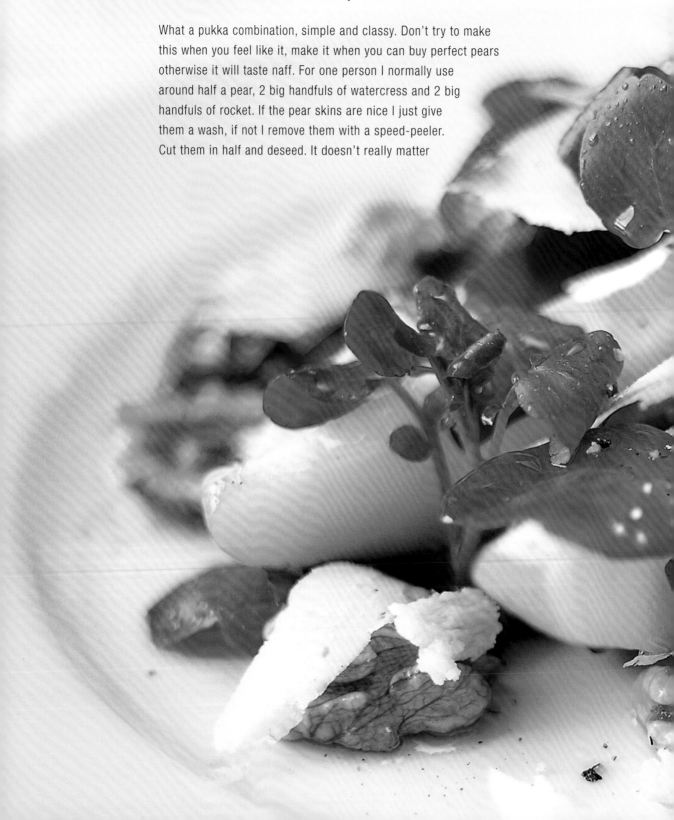

how you cut them up – sometimes in big rough chunks, maybe sliced up or even grated. Place in a bowl with the watercress and rocket – the pepperiness of the leaves works so well with the sweetness of the pear. Drizzle with good extra virgin olive oil just to coat, a small squeeze of lemon juice (because the pear juice is slightly acidic but very tasty), and season well with sea salt and black pepper. Toss all this together and serve. Shave over some Parmesan or pecorino, crumble some walnuts over and tuck in.
I love this salad with roasted meat or as a starter on its own.

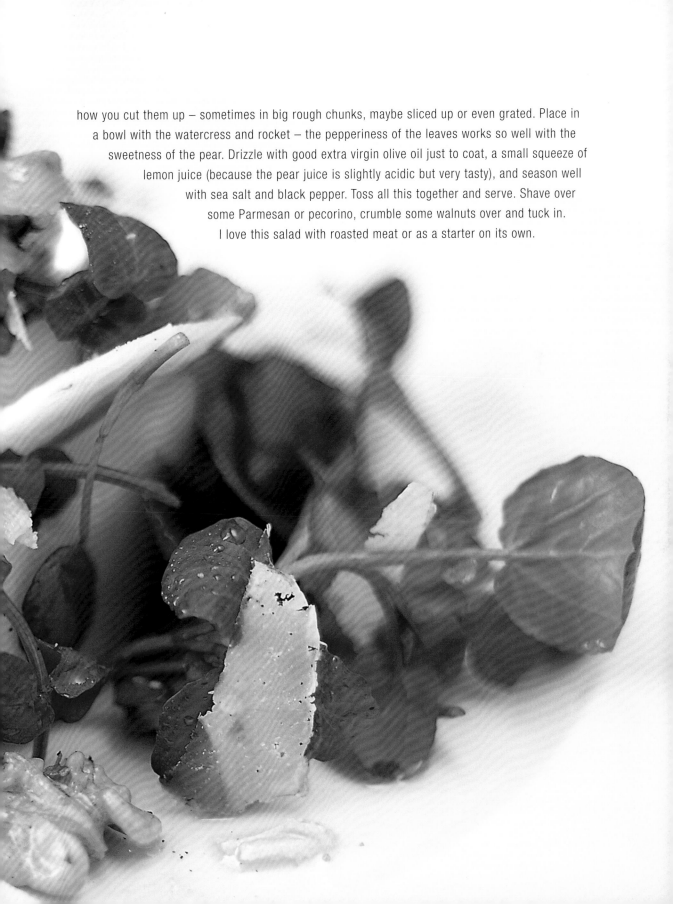

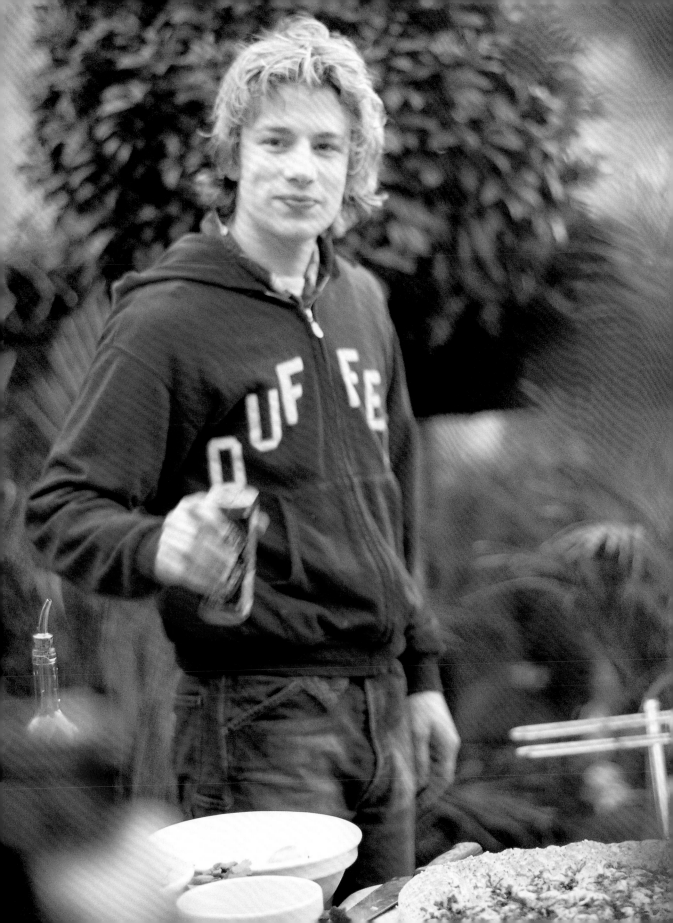

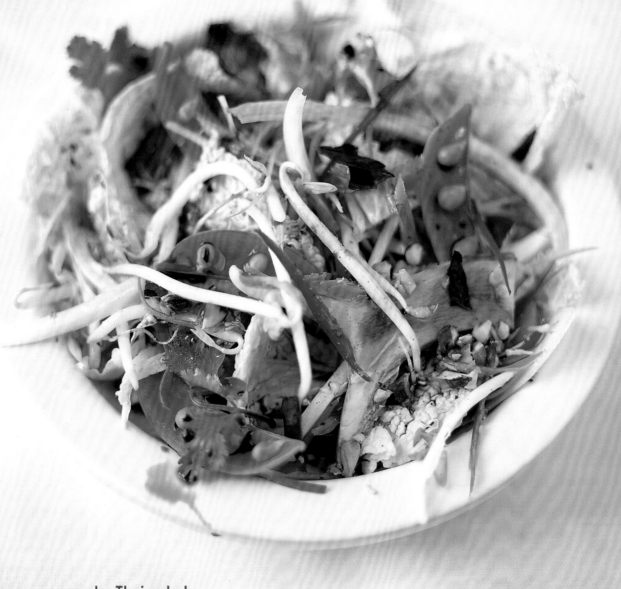

crunchy Thai salad

The thing I love about this salad is that it's so crunchy and tasty and you just know that it's really good for you. Any combination of the following ingredients is great: beansprouts (ready to eat), finely sliced green and red peppers, baby spinach, finely sliced and deseeded red or green chillies, rocket, sliced spring onions, peeled, gutted and sliced cucumbers, finely sliced Chinese or Savoy cabbage, sugar snap peas and fresh herbs like mint, basil and coriander. Dress with the Thai dressing on page 80, then sprinkle with some lightly toasted cashew nuts or sesame seeds. Fantastic. If you want to make this more substantial, toss in some cooked and chilled noodles.

mixed leaf salad with mozzarella, mint, peach & prosciutto

Try to get hold of buffalo mozzarella. I like to crumble a little bit of dried chilli over my mozzarella, but I'm a chilli freak and you may not be, so you don't have to! And use any mixed leaves you fancy.

If I make this for my lunch I'll use one nice, ripe peach, half a ball of mozzarella and a couple of slices of prosciutto. Pinch the skin of the peaches and peel from the bottom to the top, then quarter. Rip the mozzarella into small pieces and place on a plate with the peaches. Lightly season with sea salt and black pepper. Lay a couple of slices of prosciutto over the top. Dress the mixed salad leaves and torn-up mint with a little of the extra virgin olive oil & lemon juice dressing (see page 81). Throw the leaves on top. Simple!

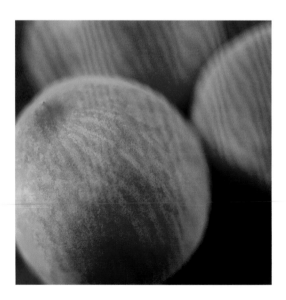

68

CALORIES	FAT	SAT FAT	PROTEIN	CARBS	SUGAR	SALT	FIBRE
412kcal	35.4g	12.4g	18.5g	5.7g	5.5g	1.7g	0.5g

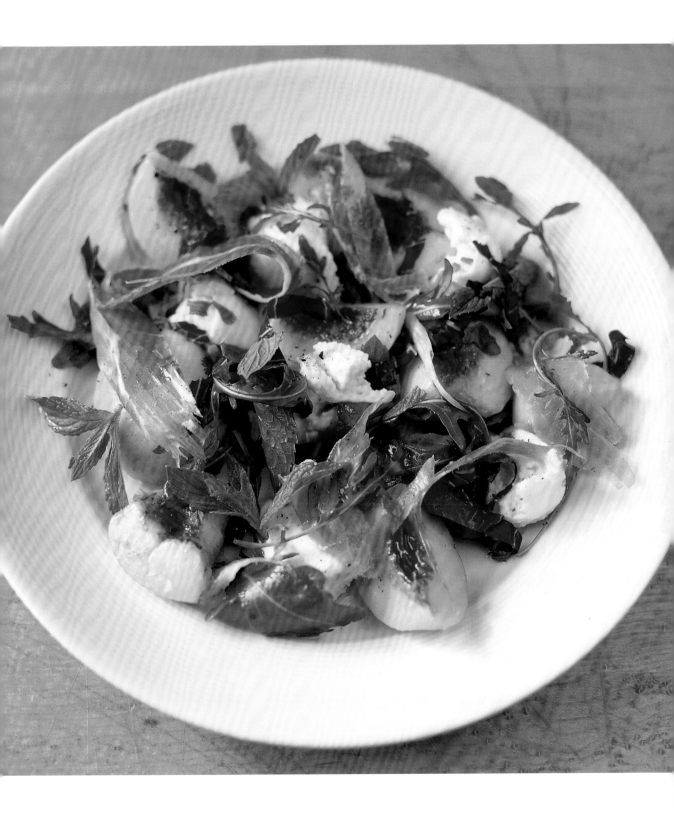

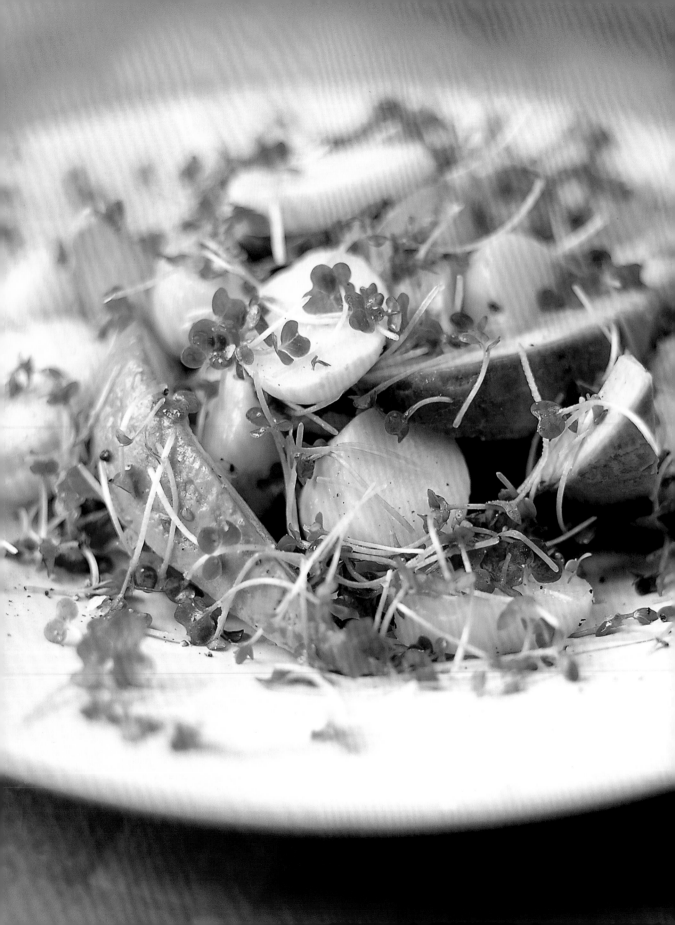

salad of boiled potatoes, avocado & cress

I had to do this salad, even though cress must be one of the tackiest things in the world. For some reason I'm absolutely addicted to it and love it to bits. This is one of my favourite combinations.

serves 4
800g new potatoes, scrubbed
1 ripe avocado
3 packs of cress
extra virgin olive oil
1–2 lemons

Cook the new potatoes in boiling salted water until tender, then drain. Slice the avocado in half and remove the stone. Peel and slice it lengthways into thick slices or chunks (however you like really) and place in a bowl. Slice any large potatoes in half – this will expose their flesh to the oil and lemon juice. If they're small, leave them whole. Add to the bowl. Throw the cress in, then add a couple of good lugs of oil and lemon juice, to taste. Season with sea salt and black pepper and toss together. Serve on a big plate, sprinkled with any remaining cress. This is brilliant with chicken, fish or as a salad on its own, especially in the summer.

CALORIES	FAT	SAT FAT	PROTEIN	CARBS	SUGAR	SALT	FIBRE
289kcal	15.5g	2.6g	4.5g	35.7g	1.9g	0.9g	3.2g

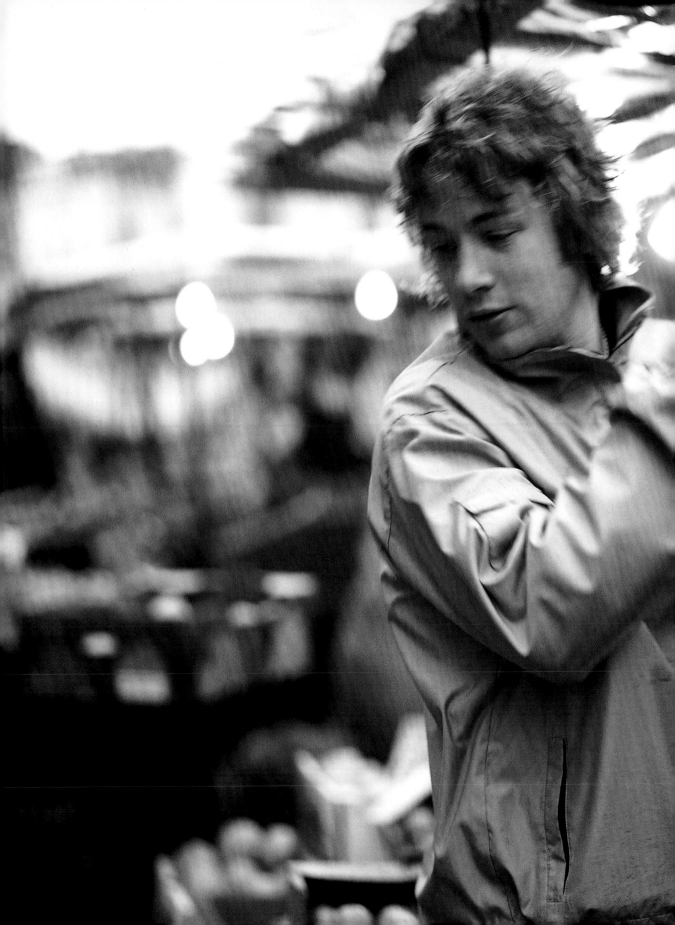

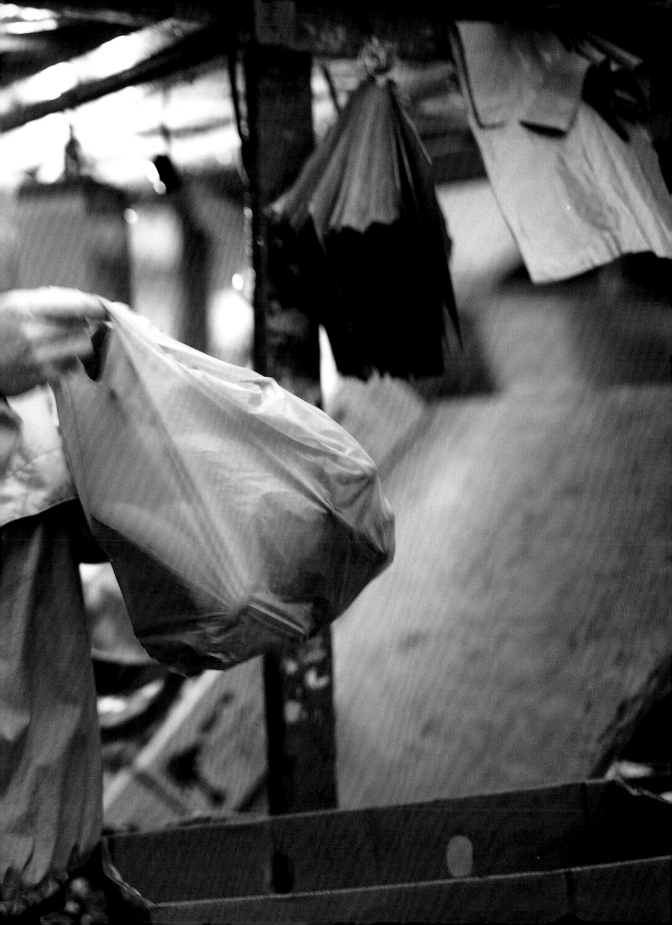

salad of marinated charred squid
with cannellini beans, rocket & chilli

serves 4–6
1kg squid, gutted and cleaned
1 × 400g tin of cannellini beans, or use 170g dried ones,
    soaked and cooked until tender
1–2 fresh red or green chillies
2 good handfuls of rocket
2 limes or 1 lemon
extra virgin olive oil

You can ask your fishmonger to clean the squid for you. Score the squid lightly in a casual criss-cross fashion. Set it to one side while you get a griddle pan very very hot – you can also use a wok or the barbecue. Season the squid lightly with sea salt and black pepper just before cooking, then put it into the pan. After a minute it should be nicely charred, so turn it over and cook for a further minute, then remove it and put it aside. Heat up the cannellini beans and sprinkle them into a bowl. Slice the chillies and add to the bowl with the rocket, lime or lemon juice and 4 tablespoons of oil, then season. Cut the squid at irregular angles and toss it in with the rest of the ingredients. A good drizzle of oil over the top will finish it off nicely.

CALORIES	FAT	SAT FAT	PROTEIN	CARBS	SUGAR	SALT	FIBRE
383kcal	18.3g	3.1g	43.2g	9.8g	0.6g	1g	4.3g

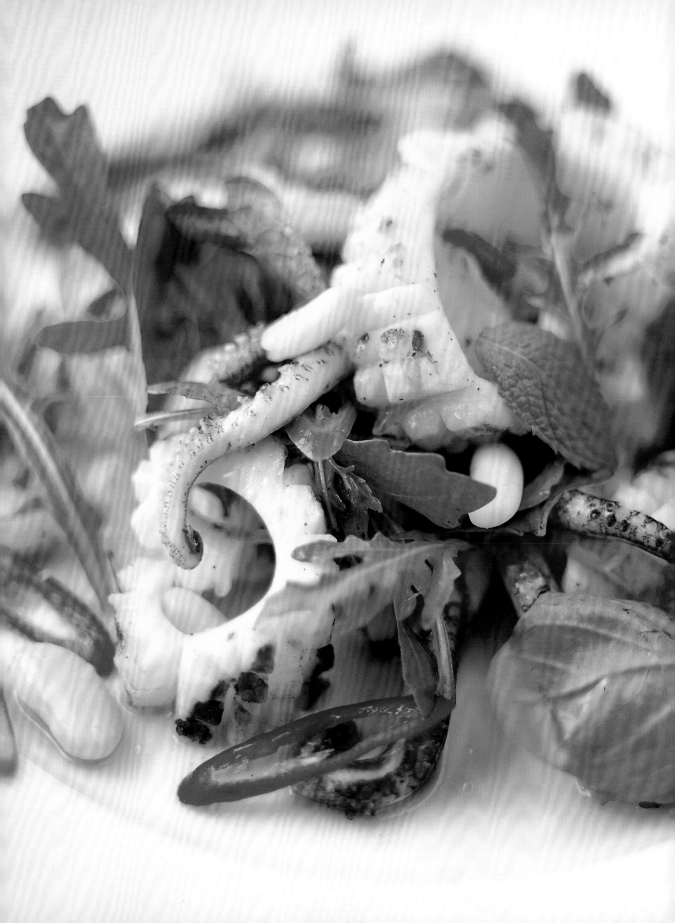

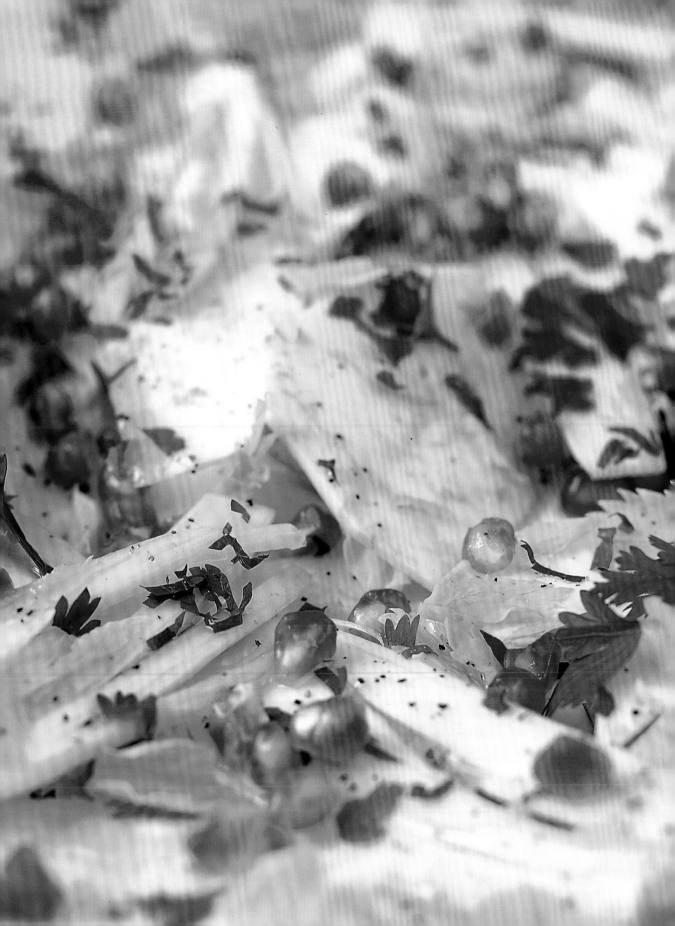

celery, celeriac, parsley & pomegranate salad

This is a really clean salad, fantastic with fish or cold meats. For it to be as delicate as it should be, the celery and celeriac should be very finely sliced. You can do this by hand using good knife skills or with a mandolin (use the guard!), which you can pick up quite cheaply. It will make the job so much easier. I normally use 1 whole celeriac to 1 head of celery.

All you have to do is strip back the celery and peel the celeriac, then finely slice. Place in a bowl with some chopped fresh flat-leaf parsley and a handful of pomegranate seeds (make sure you use just the red seeds, not the bitter yellow stuff). Season with sea salt and black pepper and dress with extra virgin olive oil & lemon juice dressing (see page 81). This salad can be dressed a little before you need it, as opposed to at the table. Place on a large plate and sprinkle with some extra pomegranate seeds. Sometimes I crumble goat's cheese over this, or some ricotta which I roll in dried herbs, salt and pepper, drizzle with olive oil and bake until golden in a hot oven.

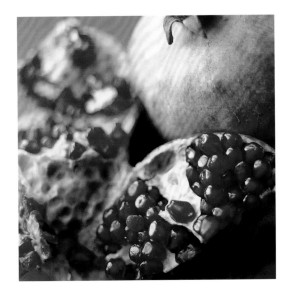

dressings

Talk about simple things making me happy. Why is it a 24-year-old boy thinks he's really clever just by making his dressings in a jam jar? I feel like a bit of a trainspotter really. It sounds almost too simple but, the fact is, we all end up with empty jam jars. Just chuck all your dressing ingredients into a jam jar, tighten the lid and shake up. Dress your salad, and any leftovers can remain in the jar, in the back of the fridge, raring to dress your next salad. And the best thing is that there's no washing up of bowls, whisks and bottles, just a jam jar.

I've found that the vinegar-based dressings taste great for a week or so, but the dressings with lemon or lime juice or dairy products in them only taste good for a couple of days. On pages 80–81 you will find six tasty dressings. Each will make enough to dress a salad for four people, but feel free to scale up, if you need more.

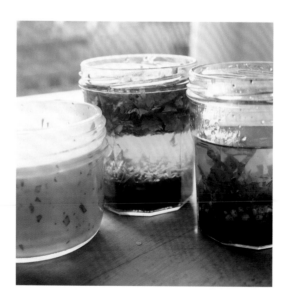

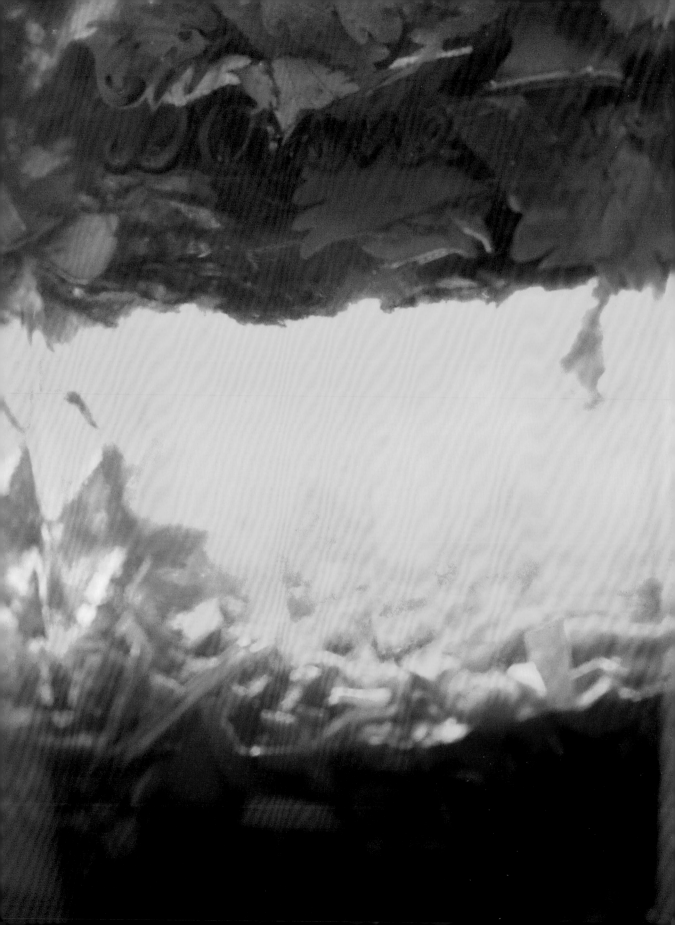

basil, balsamic vinegar & pine nut dressing

5 tablespoons extra virgin olive oil

2 tablespoons balsamic vinegar

1 good handful of fresh basil, chopped

1 good handful of pine nuts, toasted and chopped

sea salt and black pepper, to taste

CALORIES	FAT	SAT FAT	PROTEIN	CARBS	SUGAR	SALT	FIBRE
85kcal	8.6g	1.1g	0g	1.4g	1.3g	0g	0g

coriander & crème fraîche dressing

3 tablespoons extra virgin olive oil

3 tablespoons crème fraîche

3 teaspoons Dijon mustard

2–3 tablespoons lemon juice

2 handfuls of fresh coriander, pounded or finely chopped

sea salt and black pepper, to taste

CALORIES	FAT	SAT FAT	PROTEIN	CARBS	SUGAR	SALT	FIBRE
50kcal	5.4g	1.7g	0.3g	0.2g	0.2g	0.1g	0.1g

Thai dressing

3 tablespoons extra virgin olive oil

4 tablespoons fresh lime juice

1 tablespoon sesame seed oil

1 tablespoon low-salt soy sauce

1 good pinch of brown sugar

1 tablespoon peeled and finely chopped fresh ginger

½ a clove of garlic, peeled and finely sliced

1 fresh red chilli, deseeded and finely sliced

1 large handful of fresh coriander and basil, chopped

CALORIES	FAT	SAT FAT	PROTEIN	CARBS	SUGAR	SALT	FIBRE
42kcal	4.3g	0.6g	0.1g	0.6g	0.4g	0.2g	0g

mustard & herb vinegar dressing

6 tablespoons extra virgin olive oil

2 tablespoons Dijon mustard

2 tablespoons red or white herb vinegar

1 level teaspoon sea salt

1 teaspoon black pepper

CALORIES	FAT	SAT FAT	PROTEIN	CARBS	SUGAR	SALT	FIBRE
73kcal	7.9g	1.2g	0.3g	0.1g	0g	0.7g	0g

extra virgin olive oil & lemon juice dressing

5 tablespoons extra virgin olive oil

2 tablespoons lemon juice

sea salt and black pepper, to taste

CALORIES	FAT	SAT FAT	PROTEIN	CARBS	SUGAR	SALT	FIBRE
85kcal	9.4g	1.3g	0g	0.1g	0.1g	0g	0g

sweet cherry tomato dressing

6 tablespoons extra virgin olive oil

1 teacup of finely chopped ripe, cherry tomatoes

½ a clove of garlic, peeled and finely sliced

2 tablespoons red wine vinegar

1 handful of fresh basil, pounded or finely chopped

1 pinch of dried chilli

sea salt and black pepper, to taste

optional: 2 anchovy fillets in oil, chopped

CALORIES	FAT	SAT FAT	PROTEIN	CARBS	SUGAR	SALT	FIBRE
37kcal	3.8g	0.5g	0.2g	0.4g	0.3g	0g	0.1g

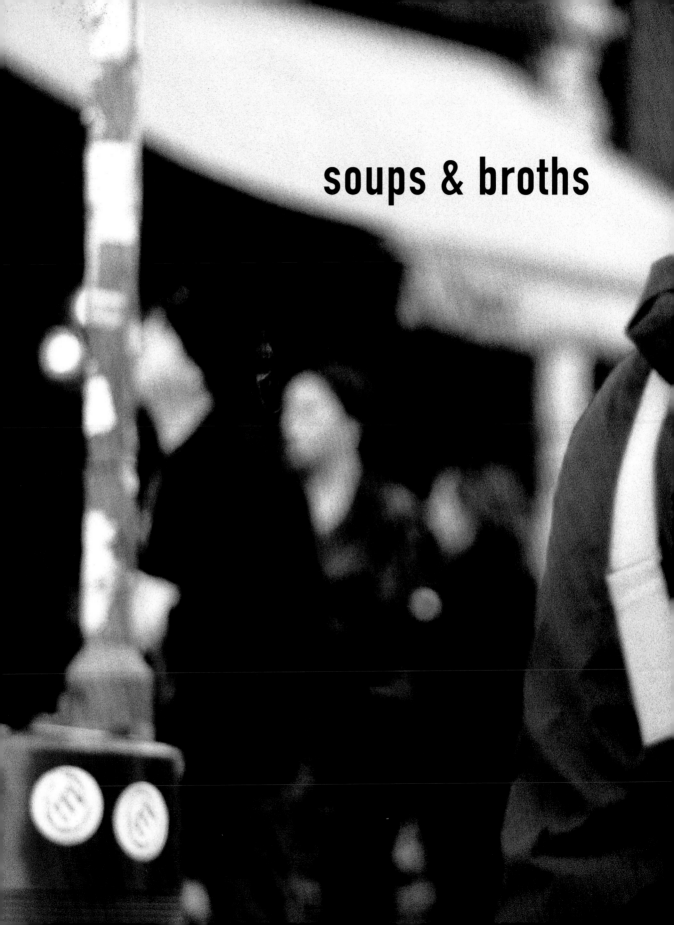

soups & broths

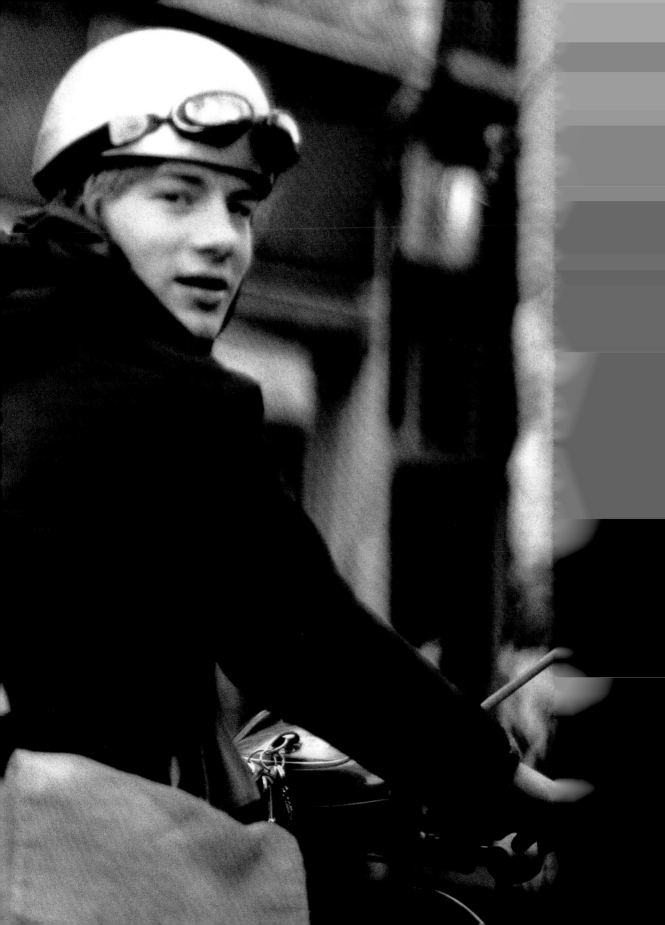

Good soups are fantastic comfort food. They're dead simple to make, but the most important thing to remember is that you must use good stock. Now before you start thinking you're going to have to be boiling things for hours, let me tell you what stock is to me at home. It's Sunday night, we've had roast chicken for dinner with all the trimmings and now I'm washing up. Two things can happen: one, I can pick up the remains of the chicken and chuck them in the bin; or two, I can throw the remains into a pot with some root veg (carrots, onions, celery and some sprigs of herbs from the window box), cover with water, then bring to the boil and simmer for an hour. There you go, fantastic tasty simple stock. I usually strain it before putting it into containers and freezing it, where it just sits waiting to be used for sauces, gravy or soups. Easy peasy. Not a stock cube in sight. If you're vegetarian then great stocks can still be made with lots of fresh vegetables – most importantly, use a handful of dried mushrooms as these will give the stock a really substantial flavour. You'll find three stock recipes on pages 275–6.

potato & Jerusalem artichoke soup
with thyme, mascarpone & hazelnuts

serves 4–6
2 knobs of unsalted butter
2 cloves of garlic, peeled and finely chopped
1 onion, peeled and finely chopped
450g Jerusalem artichokes, peeled and chopped
250g potatoes, peeled and chopped
1 good handful of fresh thyme leaves
1 litre chicken or vegetable stock (see pages 275–6)
150g mascarpone cheese
200g hazelnuts

In a large pan, melt the butter and slowly fry the garlic, onion, artichokes, potatoes and thyme. Add the stock, then bring to the boil and simmer for about 30 minutes, or until the potatoes and artichokes are tender. Blitz chunky or to a purée. Reheat, adding the mascarpone, and season to taste with sea salt and black pepper. Toast and crumble over the hazelnuts.

CALORIES	FAT	SAT FAT	PROTEIN	CARBS	SUGAR	SALT	FIBRE
714kcal	57.8g	18.9g	18.8g	33.4g	8.9g	0.3g	9.6g

Mary's Saturday soup & dumplings

Mary is the mother of my mate Kevin and her Saturday soup is famous in east London. It's great comfort food that originates from the West Indies. There are tales behind its name but basically it's a chunky, robust soup that is supposed to use up any leftover vegetables. Who cares where its name comes from – it's bloody tasty, even on a Monday, and that's all that matters! I've changed Mary's recipe to suit my taste – I'll probably get a slap for it, but that's cooking and you can do what you like!

serves 6–8

dumplings
4 heaped tablespoons self-raising flour
4 heaped tablespoons cornmeal
   (if unavailable use plain flour)
50g unsalted butter (at room
   temperature)

soup
700g stewing lamb or beef, diced
olive oil
1 medium onion, peeled and finely sliced
1 medium carrot, roughly chopped
2 tablespoons coriander seeds

2 handfuls of fresh thyme, leaves picked
2 large sweet potatoes, peeled and
   chopped into chunks
450g butternut squash or pumpkin,
   peeled, deseeded and chopped into
   chunks
450g white yam, peeled and chopped
   into chunks
1 litre chicken stock (see page 275)
1 × 400ml tin of light coconut milk
250g okra
2–3 fresh red chillies, deseeded
   and chopped

Rub the flour, cornmeal, butter and a pinch of sea salt and black pepper together, adding water bit by bit to form a stiff dough. Roll into balls slightly smaller than golf balls and put to one side.

Season the meat with salt and pepper, then brown in a large pot in a little olive oil. Add the onion, carrot, coriander seeds and thyme leaves. Shake around and soften slightly before adding the sweet potatoes, squash and yam. Turn the heat down and cook for 20 minutes with the lid on, shaking regularly. Stir in the stock, lay the dumplings on top and simmer for 40 minutes with the lid on before adding the coconut milk and okra and cooking for a final 10 minutes. Carefully season, tasting as you go. Sprinkle with the chillies before serving. Scrummy.

PS Instead of throwing away the squash seeds, roast them in a little oil and salt until crisp. Serve either sprinkled over the soup or on their own with drinks.

soups and broths

CALORIES	FAT	SAT FAT	PROTEIN	CARBS	SUGAR	SALT	FIBRE
762kcal	29.5g	15.4g	40.2g	89.3g	16.3g	1.4g	7.2g

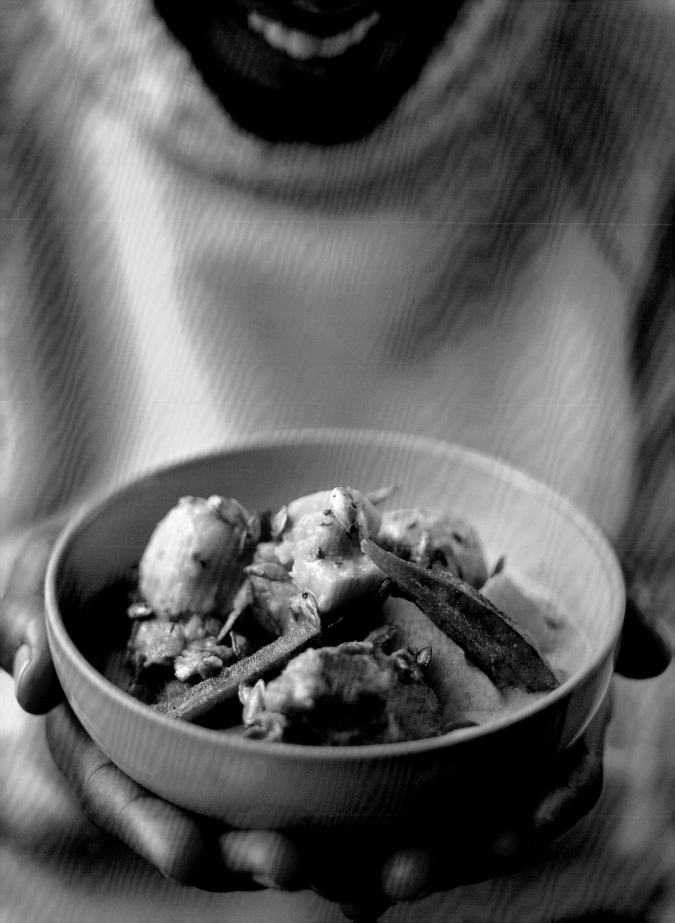

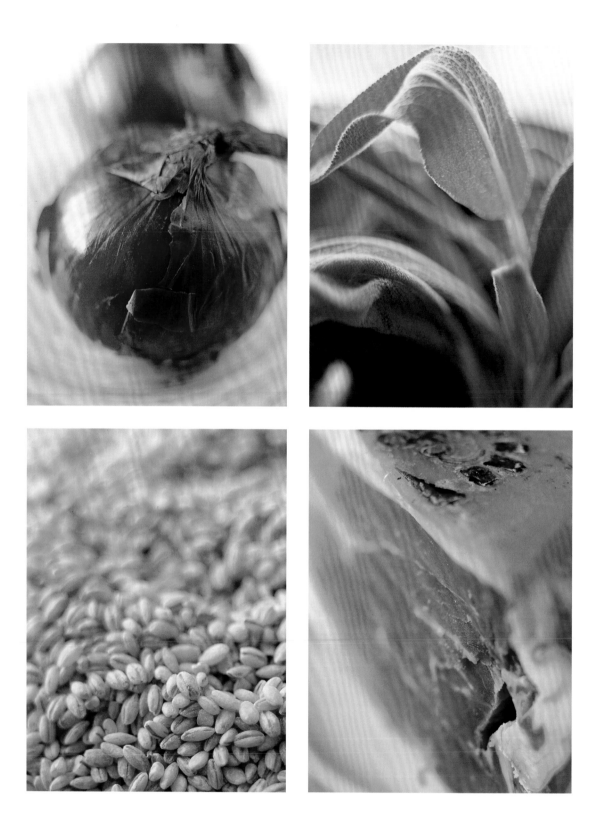

squash, Parma ham hock, sage, onion & barley broth

In Italy, when slicing Parma and prosciutto ham, the first half, which is really lean, is used in salads and meat plates. The next bit of the ham is fatty and more sinewy, lending itself to being wrapped around fish and meat when roasting. What's left of the ham is the hock, and this is great cooked slowly with beans or used in soups. In the UK we don't seem to cook much with hocks and I've found that in supermarkets they are either binned or left to one side, so ask at the deli counter if you can have one. You should pay half the price for the hock compared to the lean ham. If not, have a word with the manager. If you find you can't get hold of one, a gammon or bacon hock will work just as well.

serves 6
1 red onion, peeled and finely chopped
1 tablespoon coriander seeds, crushed
2 cloves of garlic, peeled and finely chopped
olive oil
1 butternut squash, peeled, deseeded and roughly chopped
2 good handfuls of fresh sage
1 good handful of pearl barley
1 litre chicken or vegetable stock (see pages 275–6)
700g Parma ham hock, skin removed

optional
1 handful of chestnuts, shelled
1 pinch of dried chilli
1 pinch of ground nutmeg

In a large pot, slowly fry the onion, coriander seeds and garlic in a little olive oil until softened, then add the squash, sage, chestnuts (if using) and pearl barley. Stir in the stock and add your Parma ham hock. Bring to the boil, then simmer for 1 hour 30 minutes. Remove the hock, discard the bone if there is one, then break the meat up into small pieces with two forks and leave to one side. Take half the soup and blitz until smooth. Put it back into the pan with your broken-up ham, then season carefully with sea salt and black pepper. Add a bit of chilli and ground nutmeg (if using), to taste. Feel free to loosen with a little extra stock, if needed. Delicious served with a little peppery extra virgin olive oil and some hot crusty bread.

CALORIES	FAT	SAT FAT	PROTEIN	CARBS	SUGAR	SALT	FIBRE
369kcal	16.2g	5.2g	34.4g	23.4g	9.2g	4g	3.6g

seafood broth

This broth is such a cracker. If a friend served this to me I'd be well impressed. Try it – you'll love it. I base it around mussels because they're tasty and damn good value. You can add any other seafood you like. The aïoli is not essential with this, but it is fantastic and you should give it a go.

serves 6
800g mixed seafood, such as squid, red mullet, prawns, monkfish
800g mussels, scrubbed, debearded
1 × 400g tin or 8 large ripe plum tomatoes
olive oil
2 cloves of garlic, peeled and sliced
2–3 fresh red chillies, deseeded and sliced
2 good handfuls of courgettes, finely sliced
2 large glasses of white wine
2 good handfuls of mixed fresh herbs, such as
    basil, parsley, fennel, marjoram, ripped
1 lemon

First clean up your seafood. I normally get my fishmonger to scale, gut and fillet the fish and clean the squid for me – it saves making a mess. Then all I have to do is pull the beards off the mussels. If using fresh tomatoes, score them and blanch in boiling water. Remove the skins and deseed.

   Into a very hot pan, swiftly pour 4 good lugs of oil and add the mussels. Flick the garlic, chillies and courgettes on top, shake the pan around, then add the white wine. While this is sizzling away, really squash in the tomatoes and lay the mixed seafood on top. Turn the heat right down and simmer for around 5 minutes, or until all the shellfish are open. Discard any that remain closed. Season with sea salt and black pepper and add your herbs. Serve the broth in big bowls over some toasted bread and, if you want to make it really pukka, add a big lob of garlic aïoli (see page 276) on top and a wedge of lemon.

CALORIES	FAT	SAT FAT	PROTEIN	CARBS	SUGAR	SALT	FIBRE
352kcal	17.6g	2.4g	30.1g	5.4g	3.2g	1.1g	1.1g

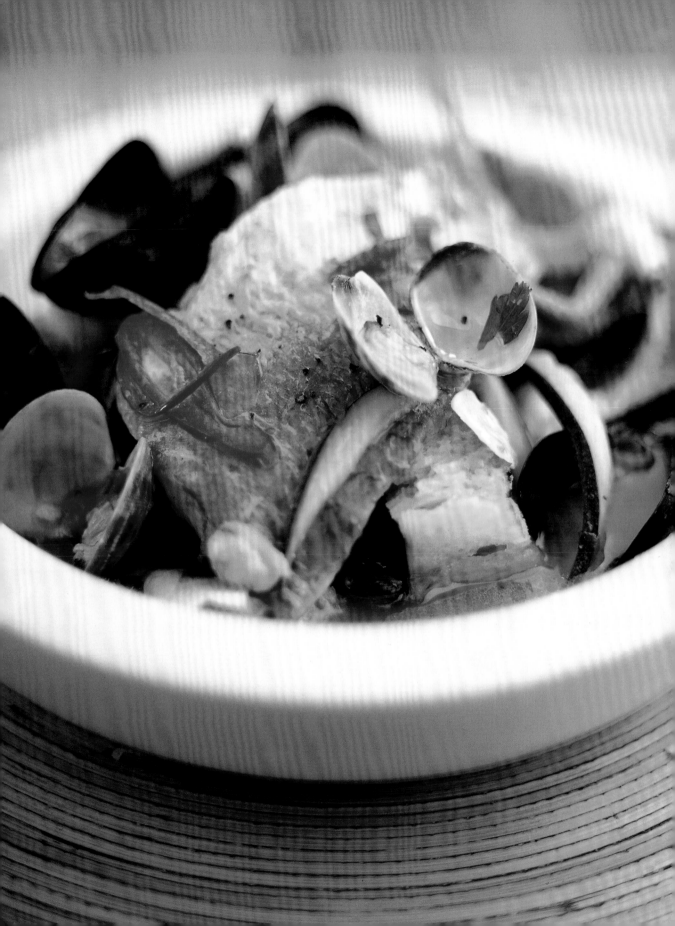

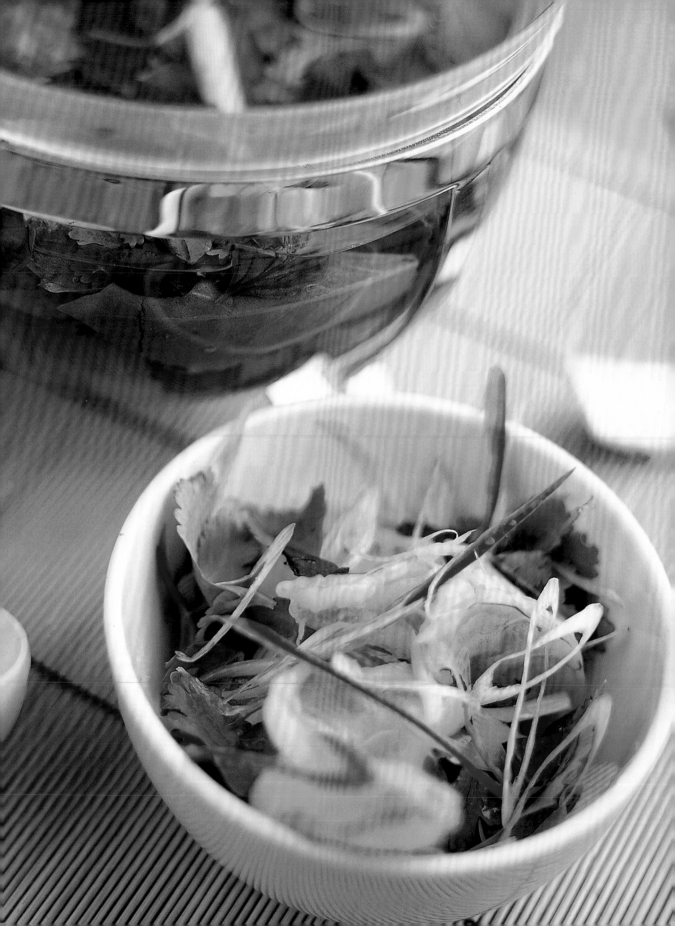

fragrant Thai broth

This is a really satisfying and almost cleansing soup. It's easy to vary this broth by using different seafood or herbs and even by adding noodles to make it more substantial. It's quite classic to have finely sliced fried onions sprinkled on top just before serving – nice idea, but another pan to wash up!

serves 4

3 sticks of lemongrass, crushed and bruised

10cm piece of fresh ginger, peeled, crushed and bruised

6 kaffir lime leaves, ripped up

1 litre chicken stock (see page 275)

1–2 heaped tablespoons sugar

4–6 tablespoons fish sauce, to taste

1–2 limes

12 large prawns, shelled, deveined and butterflied

1 good handful of fresh coriander and basil

garnish

2 fresh red chillies, sliced

1 red pepper, deseeded and finely sliced

4 spring onions, trimmed and finely sliced

In a pestle and mortar, bash the lemongrass, ginger and lime leaves. Place in a pot with the stock, bring to the boil, then simmer for 10 minutes. Taste – it should be tasty and fragrant, but slightly bland. So add the sugar and fish sauce, then squeeze in the lime juice, to taste. What you are trying to achieve with these three ingredients is a slightly sweet, sour, salty and savoury balance – but this is a personal thing, so add them bit by bit and keep tasting until you have a flavour you're happy with.

Now add the prawns to the broth and cook for 1 minute, then remove and divide between four bowls, topped with the fresh herbs and garnish. You can now finish the soup by pouring the broth into each bowl. I like a bit of drama so I pour the broth into a glass teapot, plunging in the fresh herbs. Visually this looks great, but infusing the herbs at the last minute like this also gives you a fresh and vibrant flavour. Feel free to improvise on the herbs – you don't have to stick to coriander and basil.

CALORIES	FAT	SAT FAT	PROTEIN	CARBS	SUGAR	SALT	FIBRE
108kcal	1.3g	0.4g	15.4g	9.1g	8.4g	1.3g	1.1g

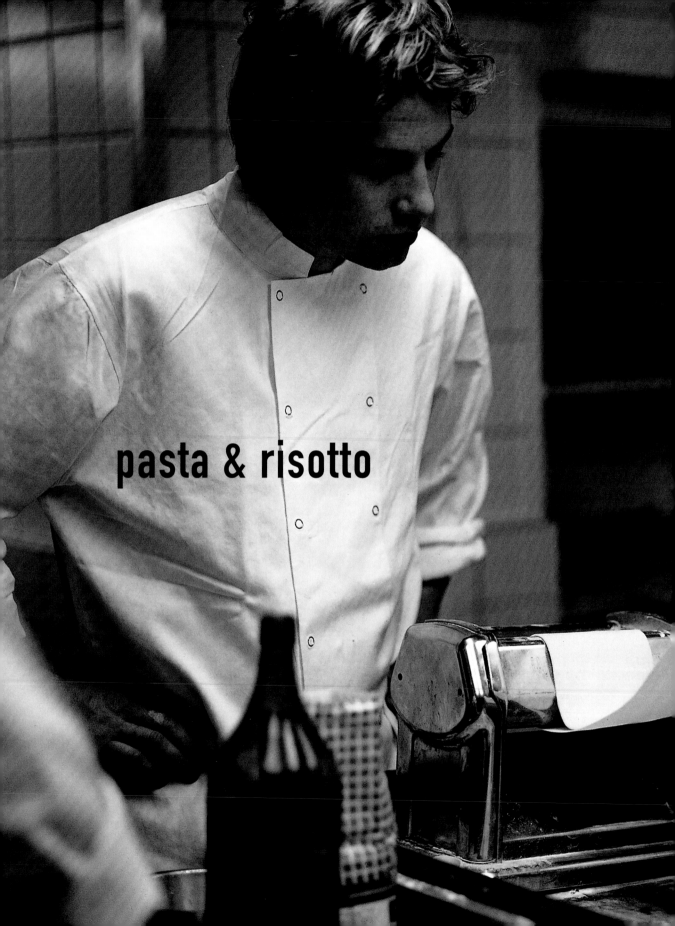

pasta & risotto

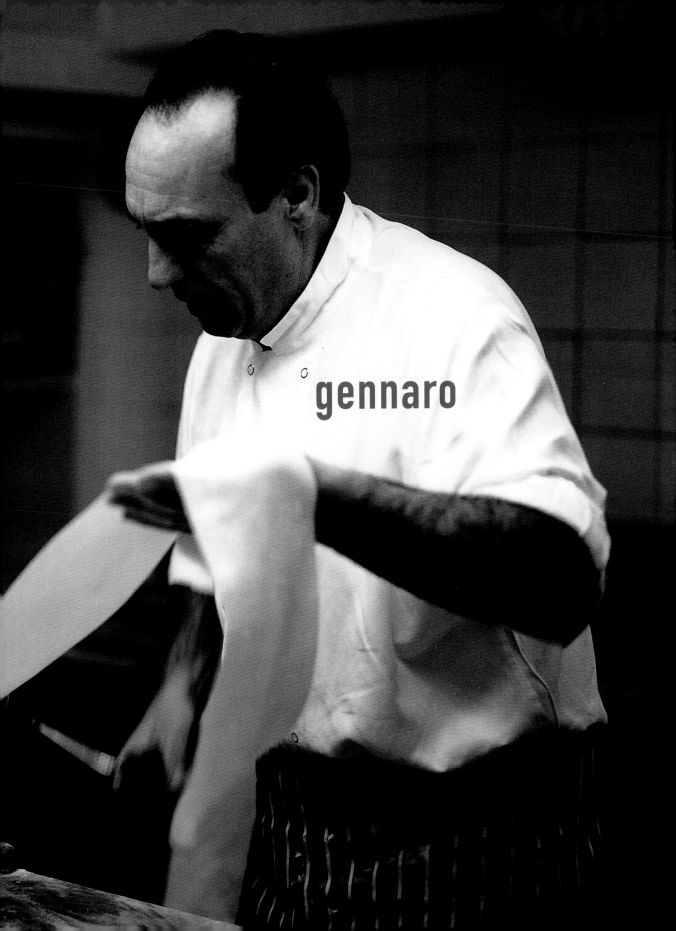

gennaro

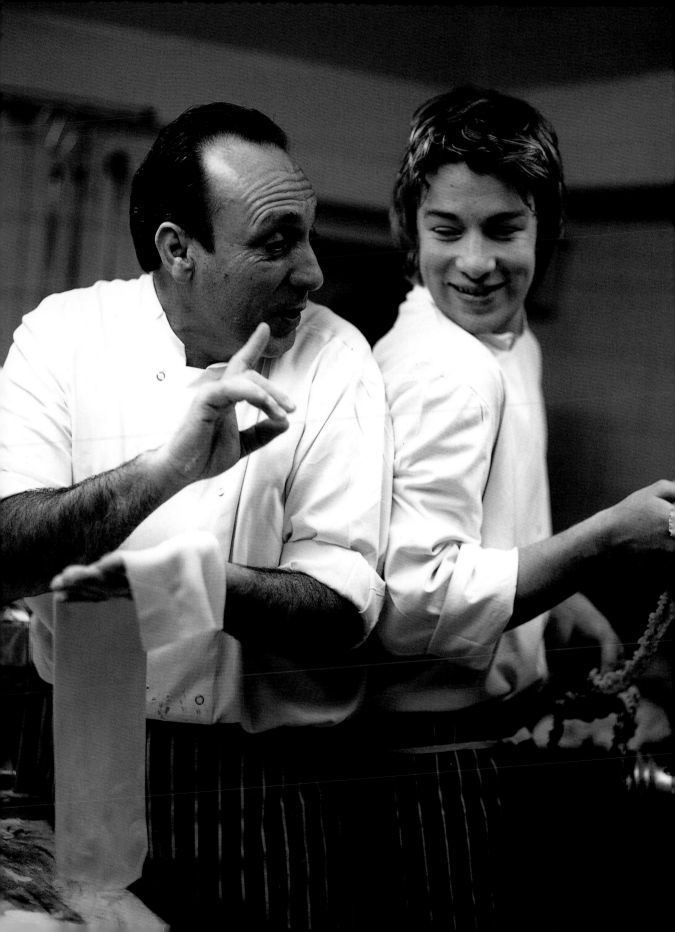

If you can crack one of these two then your mates are gonna think you're a bit clever. A good pasta dish or a good risotto just can't be beaten. We're not talking about flashy food, we're talking about something really tasty, something mouthwatering and something with a real personal touch just waiting to be eaten – that's what it's all about, whether you're in a restaurant, sitting down with your family or having a dinner party. Give 'em a try.

In this chapter you'll find amazingly quick dried pasta recipes, as well as some gutsy homemade fresh pasta for all occasions and seasons. The basic risotto recipe is fantastic, giving you the perfect creamy base, followed by some extremely simple variations – give them all a try and make up some of your own, too.

fresh pasta

Being able to make good fresh pasta is in my eyes one of the best things I've ever learnt in cooking. It allows you to put character into the pasta as well as into the sauce, making snacks, lunches, dinners and dinner parties damn handsome and wholesome. And people can tell it's homemade and just love it. You've got to try it – it will be a real asset to your repertoire. The basic pasta recipe on the next page can be made in a mixer or food processor, but I prefer doing it by hand so I can feel what's happening as I work the dough. Remember: save the egg whites that you're not using to make batters and meringues.

blinding pasta recipe

serves 6
250g strong flour
250g semolina flour (if unavailable, strong flour will do)
3 large eggs
8 egg yolks

Place both flours on a clean surface. Make a well in the centre and add the eggs and yolks. With a fork break up the eggs as you bring in the flour. Stir with the fork until you have a dough which you can work with your hands. Knead well until you have a smooth, silky and elastic dough and a clean surface. Wrap the dough in clingfilm and rest it in the fridge for a while.

I use a pasta machine to roll out my pasta into thin sheets about 10cm wide. Try to get one – they're great. They rarely break and only set you back about £25. However, you can use a rolling-pin – it just takes a little longer to get the pasta as thin. Divide your ball of dough into four pieces and keep covered. Working with one ball at a time, flatten out with your hand and run through the thickest setting on your machine. Fold in half and repeat this process several times, to give you perfect, textured pasta. Dust the sheet of pasta on both sides with flour before running it through the settings – I usually repeat this four or five times, dusting and moving the setting in each time until I have the desired thickness (normally about 1–2mm thick, depending on the type of pasta I am making). It does take practice, but once you've cracked it, you'll be knocking up pasta like no one's business. It's all about getting to grips with how pasta works. It will stay fresh in the fridge for half a day or it can be dried (see page 101) and stored in airtight containers.

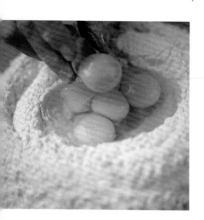 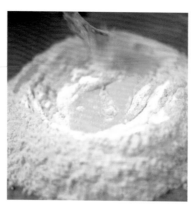 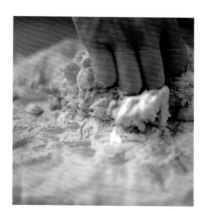

CALORIES	FAT	SAT FAT	PROTEIN	CARBS	SUGAR	SALT	FIBRE
429kcal	13.5g	3.6g	18.7g	60.6g	0.9g	0.2g	2.3g

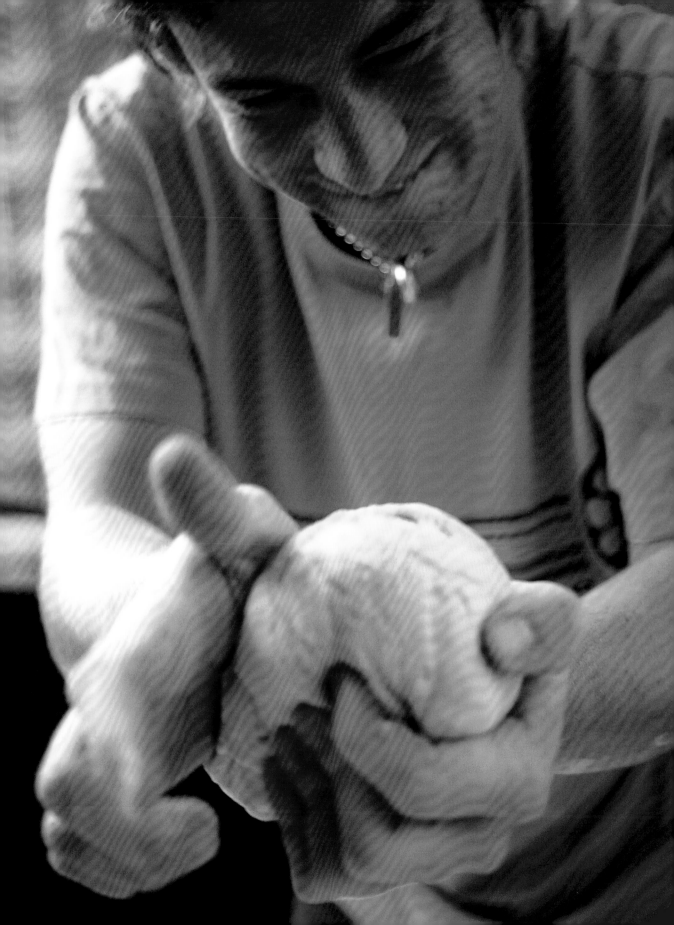

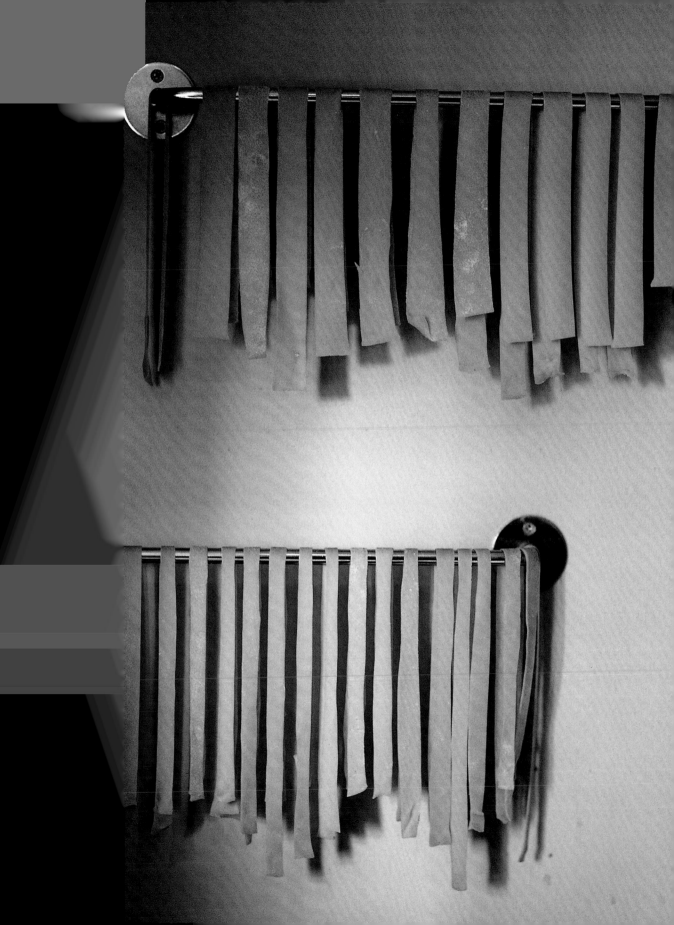

shaping pasta from a sheet

So you've got your pasta sheets in front of you – now all you have to do is shape them. Check out the recipes on pages 103–23 using stracci, pappardelle, tagliatelle, ravioli and tortellini. There are so many things you can make by simply cutting, folding or filling pasta, so what are you waiting for? Get cracking.

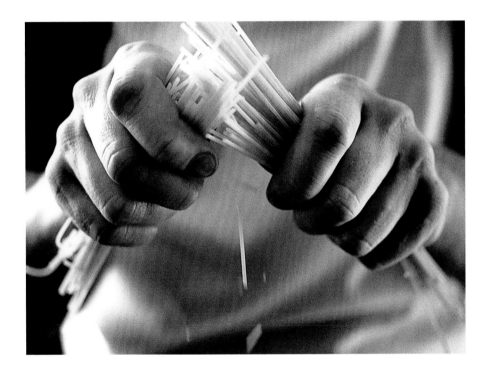

drying pasta

I generally make fresh pasta at home on special occasions or when friends are coming round. Saying that, I always tend to double or triple the recipe, making much more than I need, and I dry the rest, cutting it into any shape or size – this is great because it means I then have a supply of homemade pasta to last me, normally, a couple of weeks until the next time I make pasta. Superb.

To dry it, all you need to do is place the pasta on a rack or hang it on a coathanger or something similar for 1 or 2 days until completely dry. To test, scrunch a piece in your hand and it should crumble and snap into small brittle pieces quite easily. Dried pasta can be stored in airtight containers for a good couple of months once dried properly.

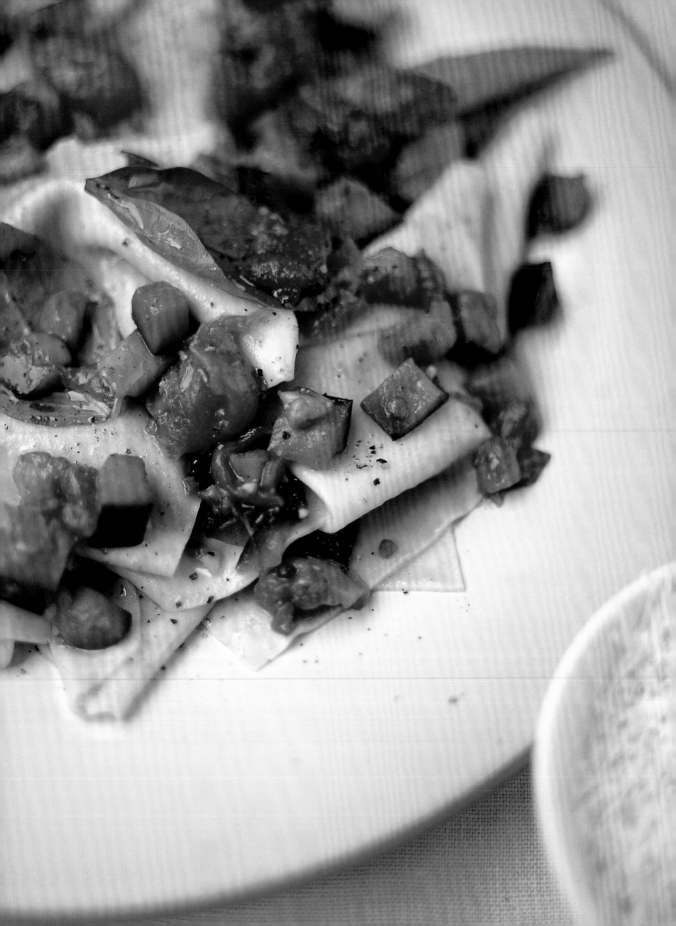

stracci

Stracci basically means 'scratched', and I love it because you can slice and scratch the sheets of pasta as you like. Cut your pieces into varied shapes and sizes with different angles and lengths (see picture on page 104). Go for interesting shapes.

stracci with spicy aubergines, tomatoes, basil & Parmesan

serves 6
1 large aubergine, cut into 1cm dice
1 teaspoon coriander seeds, cracked
1–2 dried red chillies, crumbled
olive oil
1 × 400g tin of quality Italian plum tomatoes,
   drained and chopped
2 handfuls of black olives, stone in
optional: a splash of red wine vinegar
fresh stracci: 1 × blinding pasta recipe (see page 98)
2 handfuls of fresh basil
2 handfuls of freshly grated Parmesan cheese

In a large hot pan, fry the aubergine, coriander seeds and chillies in a couple of generous lugs of oil until golden. Add more oil, if needed. Add the chopped tomatoes and cook for 5 minutes before destoning and adding the olives. Continue cooking until you have a lovely 'saucey' consistency. Season to taste at this point with sea salt, black pepper and maybe a splash of red wine vinegar. Cook the stracci in boiling salted water until al dente. Drain and throw into the sauce. Toss together, rip in the basil and serve with the grated Parmesan on top.

CALORIES	FAT	SAT FAT	PROTEIN	CARBS	SUGAR	SALT	FIBRE
564kcal	24.2g	6.6g	24.1g	65.4g	5.2g	0.6g	3g

stracci with Gorgonzola, mascarpone, marjoram & walnuts

serves 6
1 clove of garlic, peeled and finely chopped
olive oil
2 good handfuls of fresh marjoram, leaves picked
100g Gorgonzola cheese
200g mascarpone cheese
fresh stracci: 1 × blinding pasta recipe (see page 98)
150g walnuts, shelled
1 good handful of freshly grated Parmesan cheese

In a large pan, fry the garlic in a little oil with the marjoram leaves until softened. Turn down the heat and add the Gorgonzola and mascarpone. Slowly melt the cheeses – don't let them boil. Cook your stracci in boiling salted water until al dente. Now turn up the heat under the cheese – again, don't let it boil – throwing in half the walnuts. Season to taste with sea salt and black pepper. Drain the stracci and throw into the sauce. Toss together and sprinkle with the remaining walnuts and Parmesan.

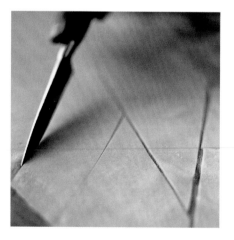

CALORIES	FAT	SAT FAT	PROTEIN	CARBS	SUGAR	SALT	FIBRE
837kcal	52.6g	19.5g	29.6g	63.6g	3g	0.9g	2.3g

pappardelle

Cut the sheets of pasta to about the length of a shoebox. Fold them over twice, making sure you have dusted them generously on both sides with flour. Now cut into slices approximately 4cm wide (see picture on page 107) and you have your pappardelle. Remember to gently toss and jiggle the pappardelle around to separate the lengths of pasta once you have cut them. This will remove any excess flour.

pappardelle with rabbit, herbs & cream

serves 6
2 good handfuls of fresh thyme, leaves picked
olive oil
2 lemons
4 rabbit legs
1 clove of garlic, peeled and finely chopped
1 small red onion, peeled and finely chopped
3 good glasses of white wine
200ml double cream
fresh pappardelle: 1 × blinding pasta recipe (see page 98)
1 good handful of freshly grated Parmesan cheese

Smash the thyme leaves with a little pinch of sea salt in a pestle and mortar, then muddle in a couple of lugs of oil and the grated zest from both lemons. Massage this on to the rabbit legs and set aside for 15 minutes to 1 hour. In a hot pan that you can put a tight-fitting lid on later, fry the rabbit until lightly golden, then add the marinade, garlic and onion and continue cooking until slightly softened. Add the white wine, cover with the lid and simmer very slowly for about 1 hour, or until tender. Continue checking to make sure that the liquid in the pan does not dry up (add a little water, if needed). When the rabbit is cooked, allow to cool slightly then use 2 forks to remove all the meat from the bones. Put the meat back into the pan with the cooking juices, add the cream and reheat. Cook the pappardelle in boiling salted water until al dente, then drain and throw into the sauce. Toss together, remove from the heat, season with salt and black pepper, then add the grated Parmesan, toss again and serve.

CALORIES	FAT	SAT FAT	PROTEIN	CARBS	SUGAR	SALT	FIBRE
842kcal	42.1g	18.4g	44.5g	63.8g	2.8g	0.7g	3.2g

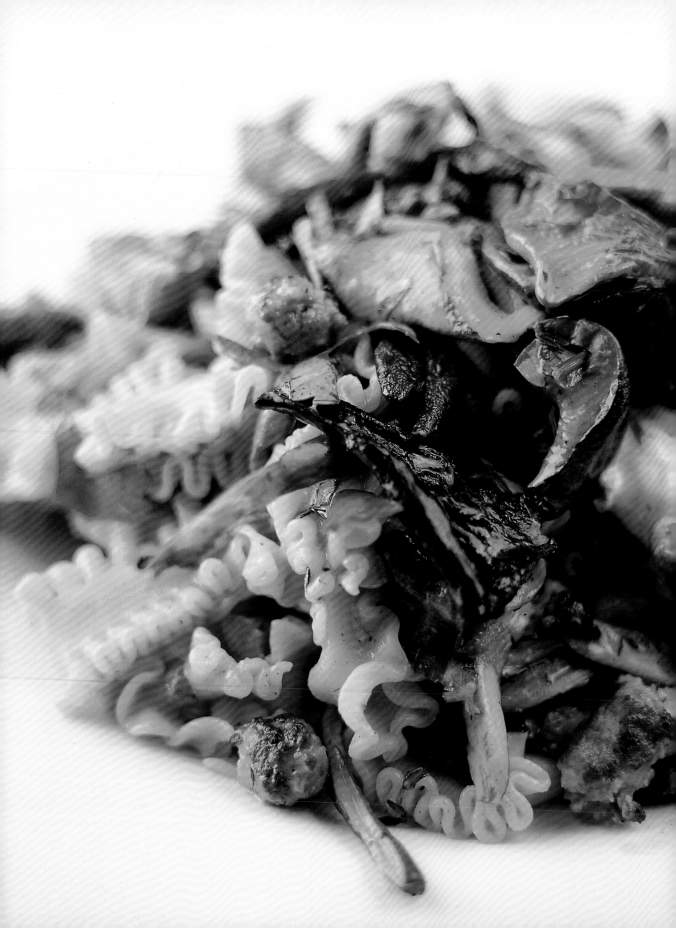

pappardelle with spicy sausage & mixed wild mushrooms

You don't have to use your own freshly-made pasta for this — you can get some really nice curly dried stuff, like the pasta seen here, which I nicked from my mate Gennaro.

serves 6

1 onion, peeled and finely chopped

1 clove of garlic, peeled and finely chopped

250g best-quality spicy sausages you can find, meat removed from skin

olive oil

2 good handfuls of fresh thyme, leaves picked

1–2 small dried red chillies, crumbled, to taste

400g mixed wild mushrooms, such as girolles, chanterelles, ceps, blewits,
    oyster, shiitake, torn

fresh pappardelle: 1 × blinding pasta recipe (see page 98)

3 good knobs of unsalted butter

1 handful of fresh flat-leaf parsley, leaves picked and chopped

1 handful of freshly grated Parmesan cheese

In a large pan, fry the onion, garlic and sausagemeat in a little oil until lightly golden. Add the thyme leaves, chillies and mushrooms. Continue to fry, cooking away any liquid from the mushrooms. Cook the pappardelle in boiling salted water until al dente. Remove the mushrooms from the heat, season to taste with sea salt and black pepper and loosen with the butter and a little cooking water from the pasta pan. Drain the pappardelle and throw into the mushroom pan. Toss together and serve sprinkled with the parsley and grated Parmesan.

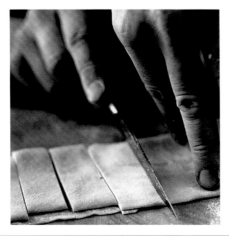

pasta & risotto

CALORIES	FAT	SAT FAT	PROTEIN	CARBS	SUGAR	SALT	FIBRE
640kcal	30.1g	12.4g	28.9g	65.9g	3.6g	0.5g	4g

tagliatelle

Cut the sheets of pasta to about the length of a shoebox. Fold them over twice, making sure you have dusted them generously on both sides with flour. Now cut into slices around 1cm wide (see picture on page 110) and you have your tagliatelle. Remember to gently toss and jiggle the tagliatelle around to separate the lengths of pasta once you have cut them. This will remove any excess flour.

tagliatelle with saffron, seafood & cream

serves 6
1 good pinch of saffron
1 glass of white wine
fresh tagliatelle: 1 × blinding pasta recipe (see page 98)
olive oil
1 large clove of garlic, peeled and finely chopped
700g mixed seafood, such as red mullet, scallops, clams,
   cleaned, debearded mussels, prawns, squid
250ml double cream
1 handful of fresh fennel tops, flat-leaf parsley or dill, chopped

Soak the saffron in the white wine. Cook the tagliatelle in boiling salted water until al dente. Put a little oil and the garlic into a large frying pan and cook until softened. Add the clams and mussels, shake the pan around and pour in the white wine and saffron mixture. Bring to the boil, and discard any shellfish that remain closed. Add the rest of the seafood and the cream, simmer for 3 to 4 minutes and season to taste with sea salt and black pepper. Drain the tagliatelle and throw into the seafood pan. Toss together and serve sprinkled with the fennel tops, parsley or dill.

CALORIES	FAT	SAT FAT	PROTEIN	CARBS	SUGAR	SALT	FIBRE
750kcal	38.9g	17.8g	36.6g	62.3g	1.9g	0.6g	2.3g

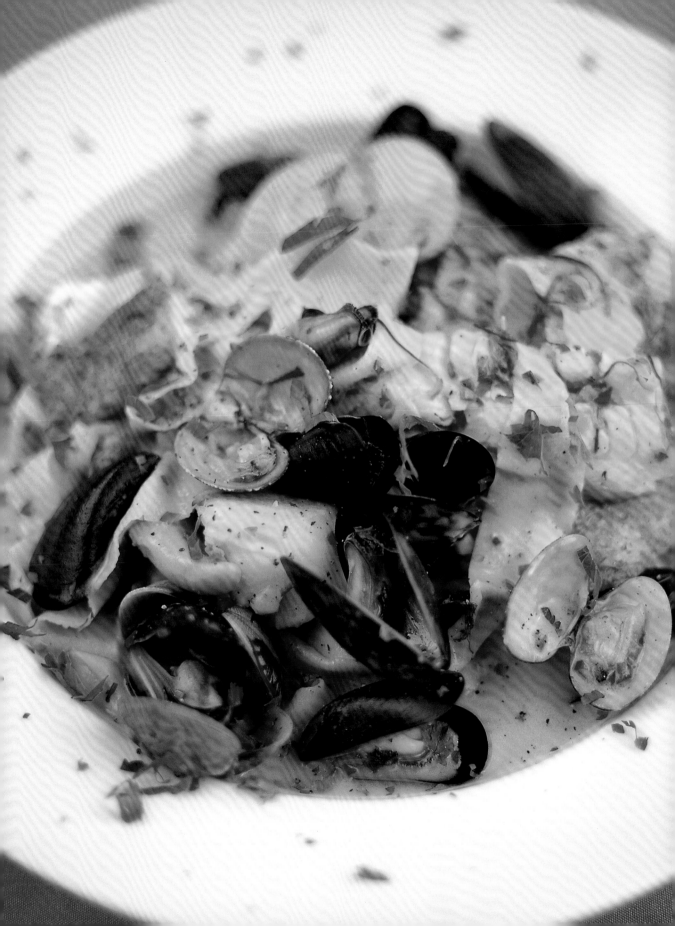

tagliatelle with tomato sauce, spinach & crumbled ricotta

serves 6
1 large clove of garlic, peeled and chopped
1 pinch of dried chilli
olive oil
2 × 400g tins of quality plum tomatoes
red wine vinegar
fresh tagliatelle: 1 × blinding pasta recipe (see page 98)
250g baby spinach
250g fresh ricotta (preferably buffalo), seasoned and crumbled
extra virgin olive oil

In a large pan, fry the garlic and dried chilli in a little olive oil until softened. Add the tomatoes, bring to the boil, then reduce the heat to a simmer – the tomatoes should remain whole until they have cooked down into a thickish sauce. Break them up with a fork or spoon. Remove from the heat and season carefully to taste with a little red wine vinegar, sea salt, black pepper and some good olive oil.

Cook the tagliatelle in boiling salted water until al dente. At the same time, steam the spinach in a colander above the pasta. Drain the tagliatelle and throw into the tomato sauce. Toss together and serve with a generous amount of spinach on top. Scatter over the ricotta and finish with a drizzle of peppery extra virgin olive oil.

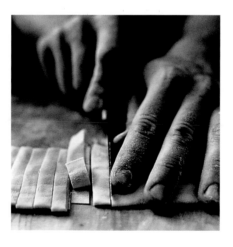

CALORIES	FAT	SAT FAT	PROTEIN	CARBS	SUGAR	SALT	FIBRE
538kcal	20.3g	6.8g	25.2g	66.5g	6.1g	0.6g	4.1g

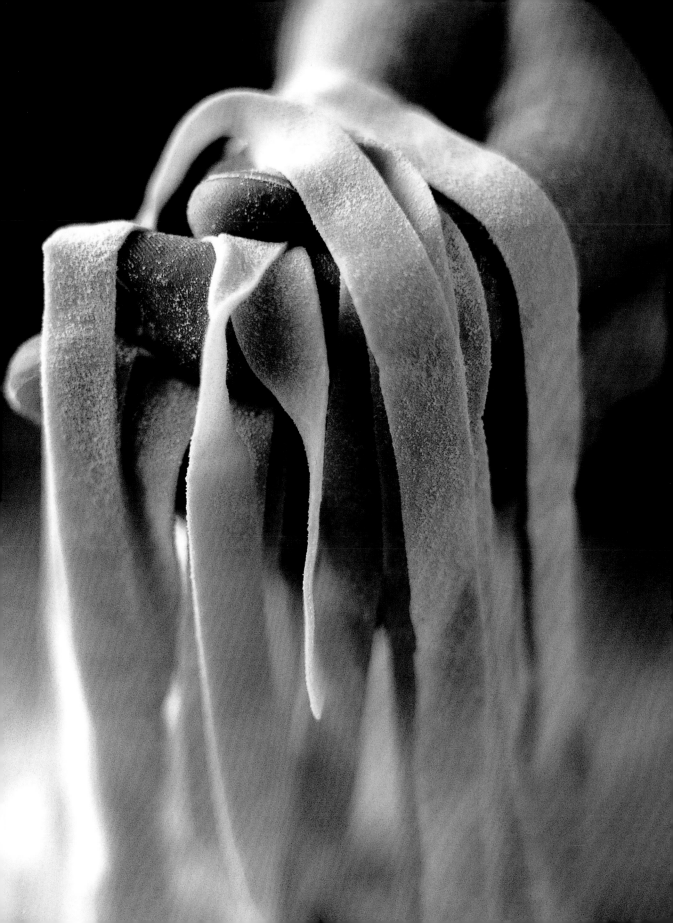

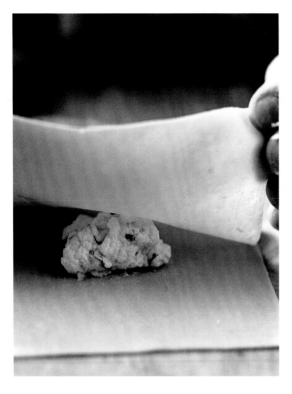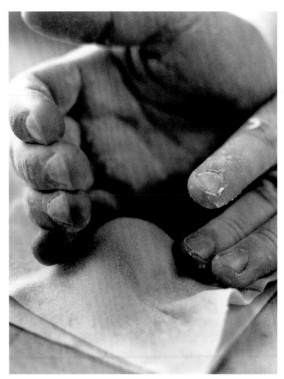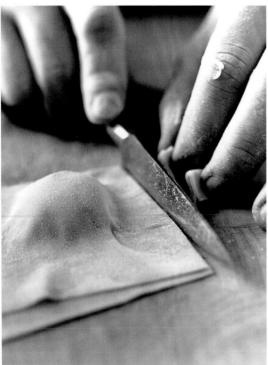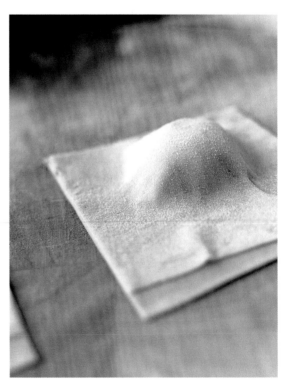

making ravioli

After rolling out the pasta sheets to about 1mm thick and 10cm wide (see page 98)
you can fill them with your chosen filling to make ravioli. Work with 1 sheet at a time,
covering the rest with a clean damp tea towel.

Stage 1

Lay a pasta sheet on a generously flour-dusted surface with a heaped teaspoon of
filling in the middle of the sheet at one end. Repeat this all the way along the pasta at
5cm intervals. Using a clean pastry brush dipped in a little water, lightly, evenly and
thoroughly brush the pasta around the piles of filling to guarantee a good seal. Place
a second, similar-sized sheet of pasta on top of the first.

Stage 2

Working from one end of the pasta to the other, push the sheets together and around
each mound of filling. Do this gently with the base of your palm, cupping and enclosing
each filling in the pasta making sure you extract all the air.

Stage 3

Cut the ravioli to shape with a knife or crinkly cutter.

Stage 4

You can cook them straight away or keep them in the fridge on a flour-dusted tray for
3 to 4 hours if you want to eat them later.

ravioli of minted asparagus with potatoes & mascarpone

serves 6

250g potatoes, peeled

700g asparagus, bases trimmed and stalks peeled (if needed)

1 clove of garlic, peeled and finely chopped

olive oil

1 good handful of fresh mint, leaves picked and chopped

1 × blinding pasta recipe (see page 98)

2 large knobs of unsalted butter

2 heaped tablespoons mascarpone cheese, lightly seasoned

1 handful of freshly grated Parmesan cheese

Cook the potatoes in boiling salted water until tender, then drain. Remove the asparagus tips and put aside. Finely slice the stalks and fry with the garlic in a little oil until tender, placing a lid on the pan. Remove from the heat, add the potatoes and mash together. Season carefully with sea salt and black pepper and add half the chopped mint leaves. Fill the ravioli with a heaped teaspoon of filling (see page 113) and cook in salted boiling water with the asparagus tips for 3 to 4 minutes. Drain and toss the ravioli and asparagus tips with the butter, mascarpone, Parmesan and remaining mint.

CALORIES	FAT	SAT FAT	PROTEIN	CARBS	SUGAR	SALT	FIBRE
614kcal	26.3g	11.2g	25.4g	71.9g	4g	0.8g	5.1g

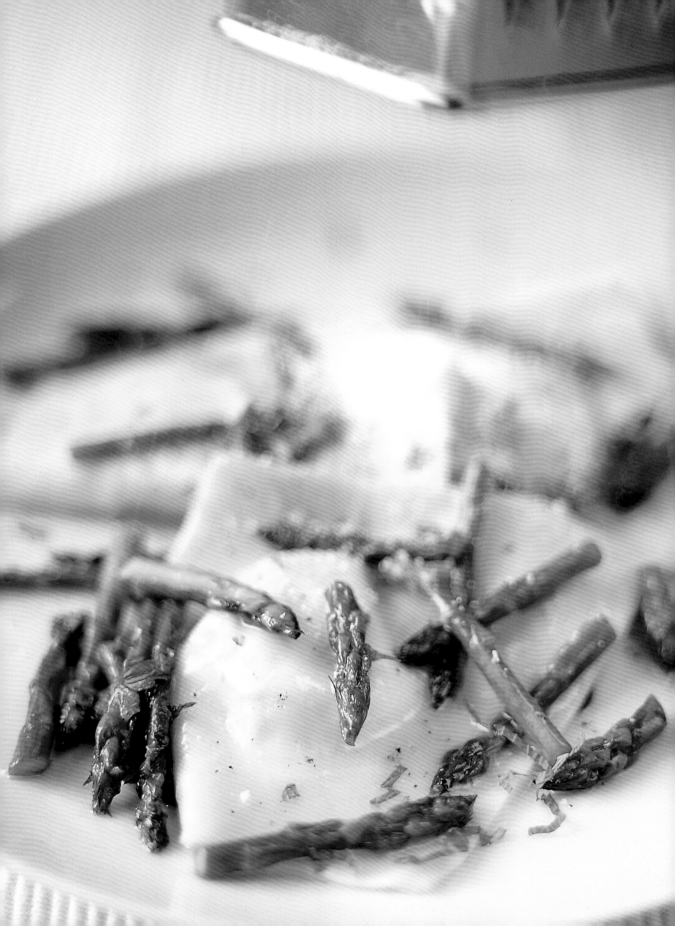

ravioli of creamed ricotta, toasted pine nuts, Parmesan & loadsa herbs

serves 6

400g ricotta cheese

1 egg yolk

2 good handfuls of freshly grated Parmesan cheese

2 handfuls of pine nuts

3 large handfuls of mixed fresh herbs, such as green and purple basil,
    flat-leaf parsley, roughly chopped

1 pinch of ground nutmeg

1 × blinding pasta recipe (see page 98)

extra virgin olive oil

With a fork, beat the ricotta, egg yolk and most of the Parmesan together until light and creamy. Toast and crush the pine nuts. Stir the pine nuts and herbs into the ricotta mixture and season carefully with sea salt, black pepper and nutmeg. Fill the ravioli with a heaped teaspoon of filling (see page 113) and cook in boiling salted water for 3 to 4 minutes. Drain and serve drizzled with oil and the remaining Parmesan.

CALORIES	FAT	SAT FAT	PROTEIN	CARBS	SUGAR	SALT	FIBRE
661kcal	33.1g	11.2g	30.9g	62.8g	2.8g	0.7g	2.4g

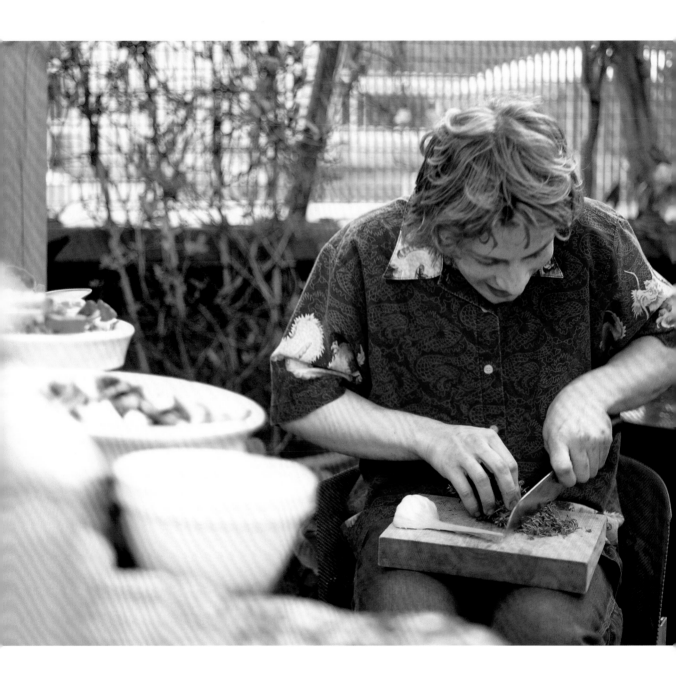

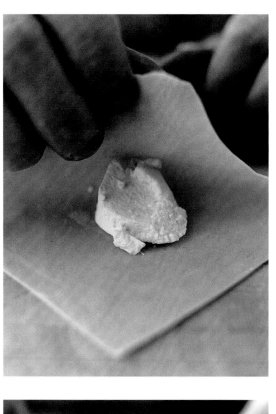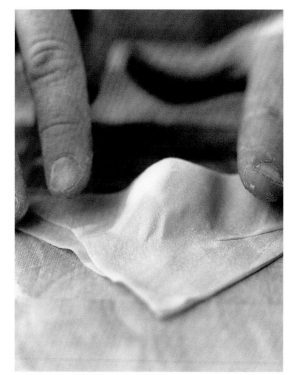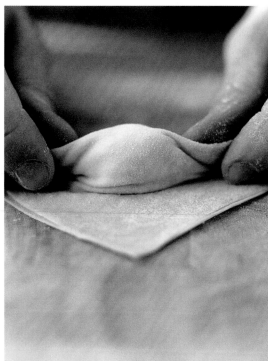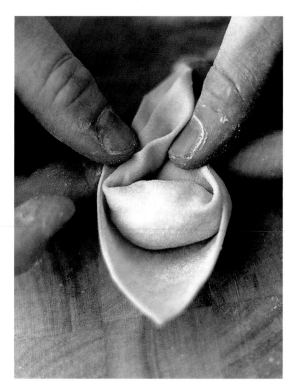

making tortellini

After rolling out the pasta sheets to about 1mm thick and 10cm wide (see page 98) you can fill them with your chosen filling to make tortellini. Work with 1 sheet at a time, covering the rest with a clean damp tea towel.

Stage 1
Lay a pasta sheet on a generously flour-dusted surface. Cut into 10cm × 10cm squares. On each square, place a heaped teaspoon of filling just off-centre. Using a clean pastry brush dipped in a little water, lightly, evenly and thoroughly brush the pasta around the piles of filling to guarantee a good seal.

Stage 2
Fold each square in half from corner to corner, enclosing the filling – don't worry if they look a bit uneven, as we want them to look homemade. Tightly seal the tortellini together by cupping your hand around each mound of filling and pressing down, making sure you extract all the air.

Stage 3
With the flat edge of each tortellini facing you, roll them once towards the tip.

Stage 4
Bring the two side flaps into the centre and squeeze them together tightly where they meet. You can cook them straight away or keep them in the fridge on a flour-dusted tray for 3 to 4 hours if you want to eat them later.

tortellini of ricotta, lemon, Parmesan & sage butter

serves 6

400g ricotta cheese, preferably buffalo
2 lemons
1 good handful of freshly grated pecorino cheese
1 good handful of freshly grated Parmesan cheese
1 × blinding pasta recipe (see page 98)
2 good knobs of unsalted butter
1 good handful of fresh sage, leaves picked

With a fork mix the ricotta, finely grated lemon zest, pecorino and most of the Parmesan together, and season carefully with sea salt and black pepper. Fill the tortellini with a teaspoon of filling (see page 119) and cook in boiling salted water for 3 to 4 minutes. Heat a large frying pan, add the butter and sage leaves and cook until the sage is crisp and the butter is foaming but not colouring. Drain the tortellini, then throw into the sage butter and squeeze over the lemon juice, to taste. Serve sprinkled with the remaining Parmesan.

CALORIES	FAT	SAT FAT	PROTEIN	CARBS	SUGAR	SALT	FIBRE
618kcal	29.5g	13.7g	28.1g	62.5g	2.4g	0.6g	2.4g

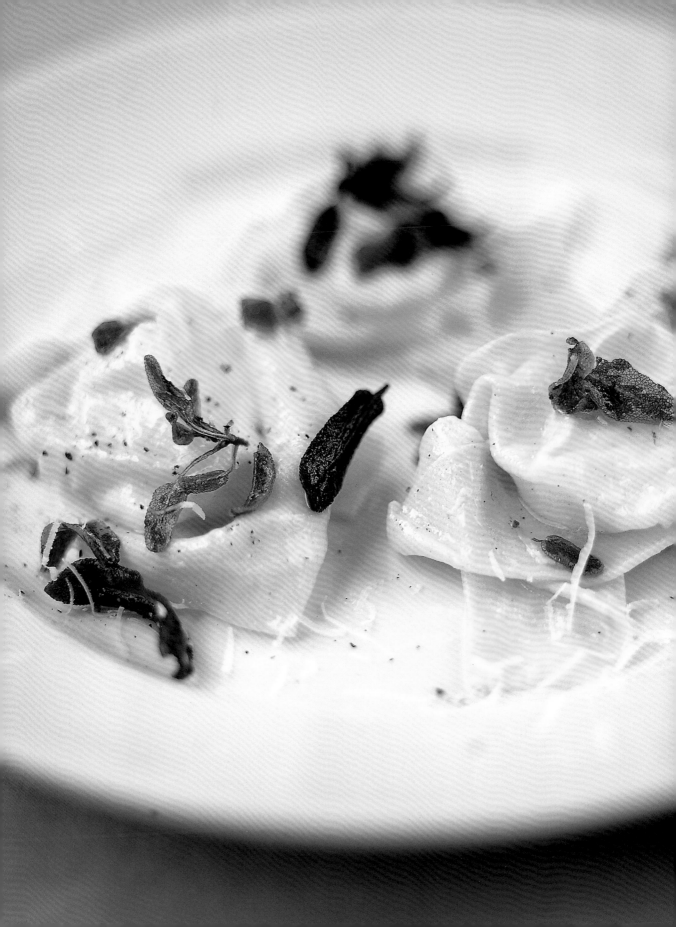

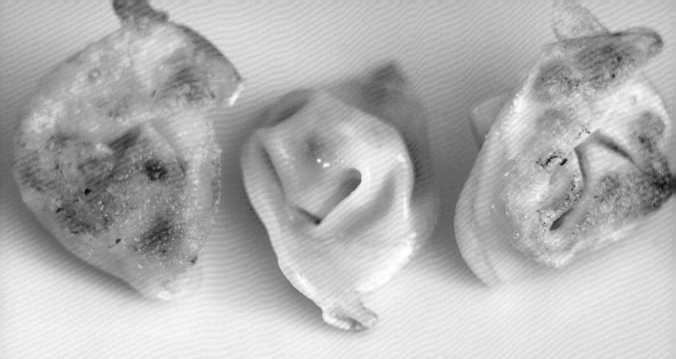

I-Thai fried tortellini of chicken, ginger, water chestnut & lemongrass with dipping sauce

This is a bastardization of the fantastic gyozas (Japanese dumplings) served at Wagamamas. They can even be deep fried for a really mad crispy texture. It's fine to improvise, using prawns, pork or vegetables in the filling.

serves 6

10cm piece of fresh ginger, peeled

2 cloves of garlic, peeled

3 sticks of lemongrass, outer leaves removed, chopped

4 chicken legs, bone out

2 good handfuls of fresh coriander

2 tablespoons sesame seed oil

1 large egg

2 heaped dessertspoons cornflour

2 handfuls of tinned water chestnuts

1 × blinding pasta recipe (see page 98)

olive oil

CALORIES	FAT	SAT FAT	PROTEIN	CARBS	SUGAR	SALT	FIBRE
682kcal	31.2g	7.4g	33.5g	69.9g	7.1g	3.7g	2.5g

In a food processor finely whiz the ginger, garlic and lemongrass. Add the chicken and whiz for a further minute. Add the rest of the ingredients, except the pasta, and pulse to an interesting, smoothish texture. Fill the tortellini with a teaspoon of filling (see page 119). Once filled, cook them for 3 to 4 minutes in boiling salted water. Drain the tortellini and place in a hot non-stick pan drizzled with a couple of lugs of oil. Fry until one side is crisp and golden, and serve with the dipping sauce.

tasty dipping sauce

You can vary this dipping sauce to your own preference, using things like kaffir lime leaves, lime juice and ginger as possibilities.

12 tablespoons low-salt soy sauce
4 tablespoons rice wine or white wine vinegar
2 teaspoons sugar
½ a fresh chilli, finely chopped
a little fresh coriander, chopped

Mix all the ingredients together, then divide between little dipping bowls, to serve.

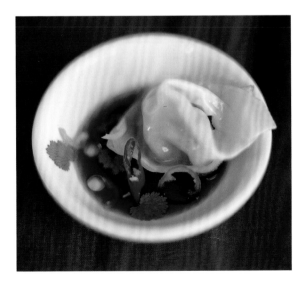

dried pasta

A lot of people think that fresh pasta is superior to dried – that's rubbish, it's just that they do different things. Dried pasta is generally made from flour and mostly water, which means that it lasts for ages and retains a fantastic bite which is great for seafood, oily and tomato sauces, whereas fresh pasta is silky and tender and suits being stuffed and served with creamy and buttery sauces. Here are some of my favourite dried pasta recipes.

spaghetti with squashed olives, tomatoes, garlic, olive oil & chopped rocket

serves 6
1 good handful of olives, stone in
olive oil
1 clove of garlic, peeled and finely chopped
1 small dried chilli, to taste
3 good handfuls of ripe cherry or plum tomatoes,
   deseeded and roughly chopped
450g dried spaghetti
3 good handfuls of rocket, roughly chopped

Destone and tear up the olives. Put a couple of good lugs of oil into a large hot frying pan and fry the garlic and chilli for 30 seconds before adding the tomatoes and olives. Toss together and allow to cook for a further 4 to 6 minutes. Meanwhile, cook the spaghetti in boiling salted water until al dente. The tomatoes will thicken into a lovely sauce with some nice fresh chunks in it as well. Drain the spaghetti and throw it into the sauce. Season to taste with sea salt and black pepper.

Add the chopped rocket, toss quickly, and serve immediately in a big bowl. Don't waste any time – get it on the table, let people help themselves and have a nice big green salad, a bit of bread and some wine. Lovely, fantastic.

CALORIES	FAT	SAT FAT	PROTEIN	CARBS	SUGAR	SALT	FIBRE
306kcal	5.3g	0.8g	9.6g	58.8g	3g	0.2g	1g

spaghetti with olive oil, garlic, chilli & parsley

serves 6
450g dried spaghetti
1 large clove of garlic, peeled and finely chopped
olive oil
1–2 fresh red chillies, deseeded and finely chopped
1 good handful of fresh flat-leaf parsley, finely chopped

While cooking the spaghetti in boiling salted water until al dente, slowly fry the garlic in a couple of good lugs of oil until softened. Add the chillies, drained spaghetti and parsley. Toss to coat, season with sea salt and black pepper and serve.

CALORIES	FAT	SAT FAT	PROTEIN	CARBS	SUGAR	SALT	FIBRE
290kcal	4.6g	0.7g	8.7g	57.1g	1.7g	0.4g	0g

spaghetti with red onions, sun-dried tomatoes, balsamic vinegar & basil

serves 6
450g dried spaghetti
1 red onion, peeled and finely chopped
olive oil
2 handfuls of sun-dried tomatoes in oil, chopped
3 tablespoons balsamic vinegar
2 handfuls of fresh basil, torn
1 small handful of freshly grated Parmesan or pecorino cheese

While cooking the spaghetti in boiling salted water until al dente, slowly fry the onion in a couple of lugs of oil until softened. Stir in the tomatoes and vinegar, and throw in the drained spaghetti. Season with sea salt and black pepper and toss together with the basil. Serve with the grated Parmesan or pecorino.

CALORIES	FAT	SAT FAT	PROTEIN	CARBS	SUGAR	SALT	FIBRE
345kcal	6.7g	1.4g	10.8g	63.7g	6.4g	1g	1g

spaghetti with anchovies, dried chilli & pangrattato

Pangrattato is great. It's basically fried or toasted breadcrumbs in garlic oil. In Italy, pangrattato was once used as a substitute for Parmesan, which some people couldn't afford. It gives a dish an excellent texture and crunch and, if made well, great flavour.

serves 6
450g dried spaghetti
4 tablespoons olive oil
2 cloves of garlic, peeled and finely chopped
16 anchovy fillets, in oil
2 lemons
2 small dried red chillies, crumbled

pangrattato
6 tablespoons olive oil
1 clove of garlic, peeled and sliced
1 good handful of fresh thyme, leaves picked
200g fresh breadcrumbs

First make the pangrattato. Put the oil into a hot thick-bottomed pan. Add the garlic, thyme and breadcrumbs; they will fry and begin to toast. Stir for a couple of minutes, or until the breadcrumbs are really crisp and golden. Season with a little sea salt and black pepper and drain on kitchen paper.

Cook the spaghetti in boiling salted water until al dente. While it is cooking, put the oil and garlic into a pan and heat gently. As the garlic begins to soften, lay the anchovy fillets over the top. After a minute you will see them begin to melt. Squeeze in the lemon juice and sprinkle in the dried chillies. Drain the spaghetti and throw it into the sauce. Taste a bit of pasta – it may need a little more lemon juice and a little extra seasoning. Serve straight away, sprinkled really generously with the pangrattato.

CALORIES	FAT	SAT FAT	PROTEIN	CARBS	SUGAR	SALT	FIBRE
595kcal	24.3g	3.5g	14.8g	82.1g	4.4g	1.6g	2g

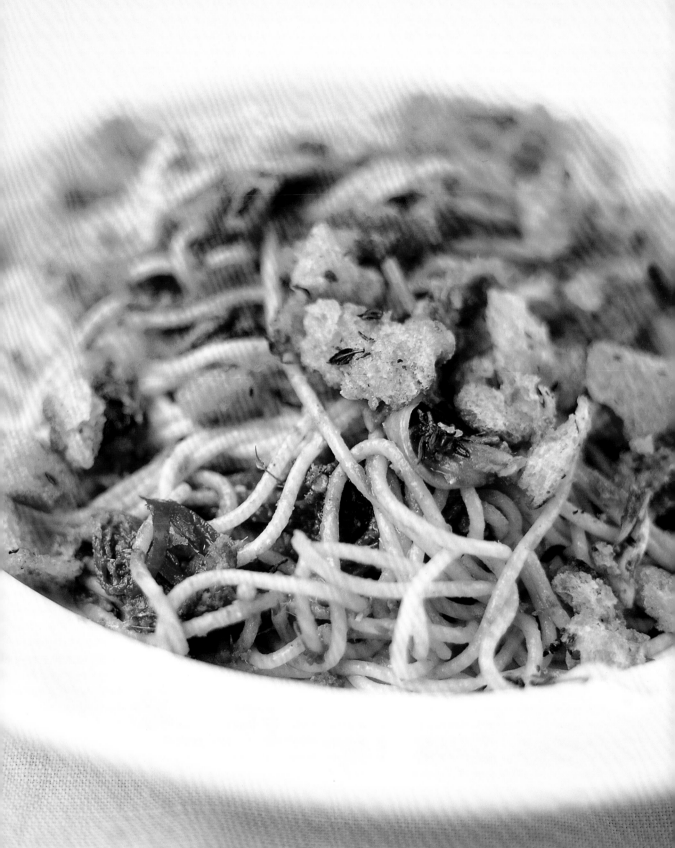

linguine with pancetta, olive oil, chilli, clams & white wine

serves 6
450g dried linguine
olive oil
4 rashers of pancetta or dry-cured smoked bacon, thinly sliced
1 large clove of garlic, peeled and finely chopped
1–2 dried red chillies, crumbled
700g clams
2 glasses of white wine
1 good handful of fresh flat-leaf parsley, roughly chopped

Cook the linguine in boiling salted water until al dente. Meanwhile, fry the pancetta in a couple of good lugs of oil in a hot pan until golden, then add the garlic and chillies. Soften slightly and add the clams. Stir, then pour in the white wine. Cover with a lid and cook for a further couple of minutes, or until the clams have opened – discard any that remain closed. Remove from the heat and add the drained linguine. Stir in the parsley, taste and season with sea salt and black pepper, and serve with all the cooking juices.

CALORIES	FAT	SAT FAT	PROTEIN	CARBS	SUGAR	SALT	FIBRE
426kcal	6.6g	1.1g	23.8g	60.2g	2g	0.3g	0.1g

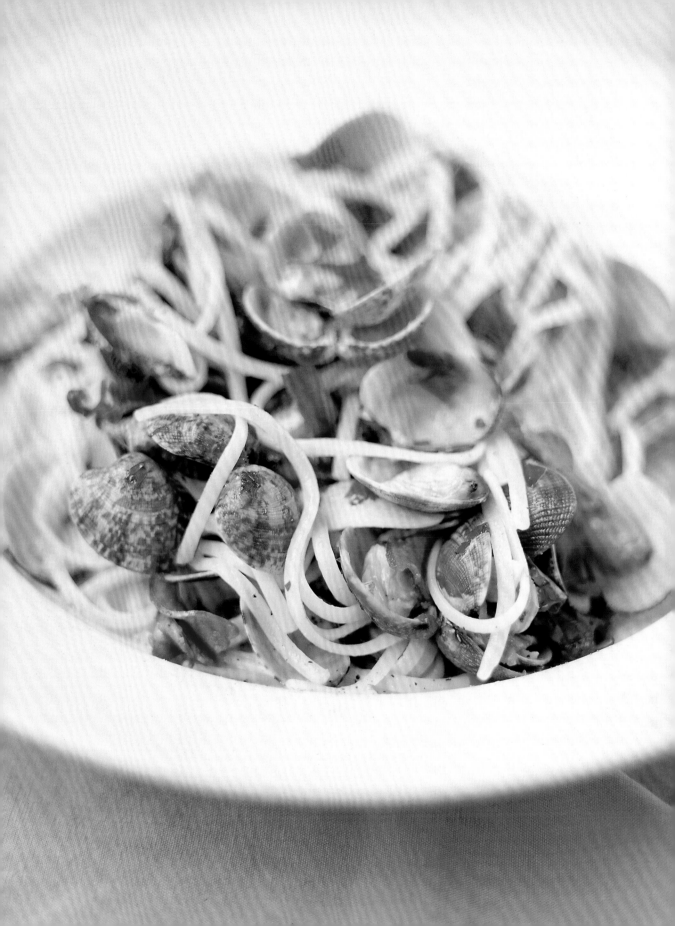

linguine puttanesca

serves 6
450g dried linguine
3 cloves of garlic, peeled and finely chopped
2–3 small dried red chillies, crumbled
1 teaspoon dried oregano
olive oil
2 × 400g tins of quality plum tomatoes, drained and chopped
2 handfuls of big black olives, stone in
1 handful of baby capers, soaked in water and drained
12 anchovy fillets, in oil, roughly chopped
1 good handful of fresh basil
extra virgin olive oil

Cook the linguine in boiling salted water until al dente. Meanwhile, fry the garlic, chillies and oregano in a little olive oil until slightly softened. Add the tomatoes and bring to a simmer. Destone and add the olives, add the capers and anchovies, then continue to cook another 4 or 5 minutes, or until you have a lovely sauce consistency. Remove from the heat, throw the drained linguine into the sauce and toss together. Rip over all the basil, taste and season with sea salt and black pepper, and drizzle with good extra virgin olive oil.

CALORIES	FAT	SAT FAT	PROTEIN	CARBS	SUGAR	SALT	FIBRE
324kcal	4.9g	0.7g	11.9g	62.3g	6.7g	1.6g	1.3g

farfalle with broccoli, anchovies & chilli

serves 6
2 heads of broccoli
1 large clove of garlic, peeled and finely chopped
15 anchovy fillets, in oil
2–3 small dried red chillies, crumbled
olive oil
450g dried farfalle
1 handful of pine nuts

Remove the buds from the broccoli, and trim, peel and finely chop the stalks. In a pan, fry the garlic, anchovies, chillies and all the broccoli very slowly in a couple of lugs of oil for about 15 minutes with the lid on, adding a little water, if needed. Feel free to mash some of the broccoli up as it cooks, giving you a chunky puréed sauce. Season to taste with sea salt and black pepper. Cook the farfalle in boiling salted water until al dente. Throw the drained farfalle into the sauce, adding a little starchy cooking water to loosen if necessary. Toast and throw in the pine nuts just before serving.

CALORIES	FAT	SAT FAT	PROTEIN	CARBS	SUGAR	SALT	FIBRE
365kcal	9.3g	1.1g	14.8g	59.8g	3.4g	1.2g	3.4g

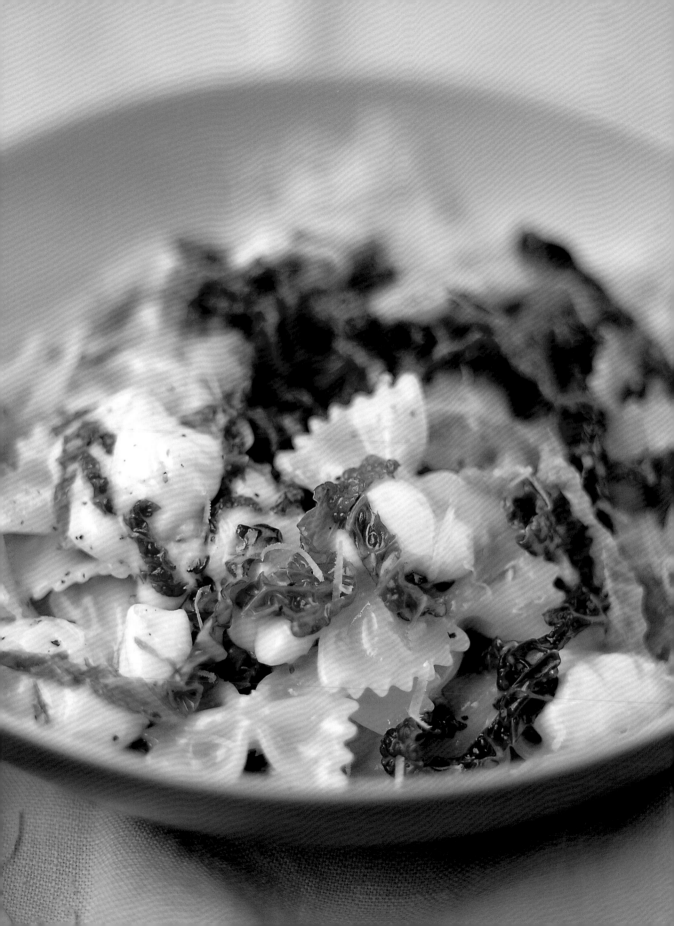

farfalle with Savoy cabbage, pancetta, thyme & mozzarella

serves 6

10 rashers of pancetta or dry-cured smoked
 streaky bacon, thinly sliced
olive oil
1 clove of garlic, peeled and finely chopped
1 good handful of fresh thyme, leaves picked
1 large Savoy cabbage (outer leaves removed),
 quartered, cored and finely sliced
1 handful of freshly grated Parmesan cheese
450g dried farfalle
extra virgin olive oil
2 handfuls of pine nuts, lightly toasted
200g buffalo mozzarella, cut into 1cm dice

Fry the pancetta in a little olive oil in a hot pan until lightly golden. Add the garlic and
thyme leaves and soften. Add the Savoy cabbage and Parmesan, then stir and cover
with a lid. Cook for a further 5 minutes, shaking every now and again, while you cook
the farfalle in boiling salted water until al dente. When the cabbage is nice and tender,
season with sea salt and black pepper and loosen with some nice peppery extra virgin
olive oil. Throw the drained farfalle into the cabbage. Toast the pine nuts and add at
the last minute with the mozzarella. Serve immediately.

CALORIES	FAT	SAT FAT	PROTEIN	CARBS	SUGAR	SALT	FIBRE
533kcal	23.4g	9.7g	22.1g	62.2g	6.7g	1.2g	3.7g

return of the risotto

I think this is the best basic risotto recipe you will come across – you will find it really easy. I assure you that once you've got the knack you'll carry on making it all the time and it won't let you down. You can so easily enhance it by adding different seasonal ingredients. So here's the basic risotto, which will give you an amazingly creamy base, followed by some simple recipes to take the dish in completely different directions.

basic risotto recipe

serves 6

1 litre stock (chicken, fish or vegetable as appropriate – see pages 275–6)
1 tablespoon olive oil
2 medium onions or 3 shallots, peeled and finely chopped
2 cloves of garlic, peeled and finely chopped
½ a head of celery, finely chopped
400g risotto rice
2 wine glasses of dry white vermouth (dry Martini or
    Noilly Prat) or dry white wine
70g unsalted butter
100g freshly grated Parmesan cheese

Stage 1
Heat the stock. In a separate pan, heat the oil, add the onions or shallots, garlic and celery, and fry slowly for about 4 minutes. When the vegetables have softened, add the rice and turn up the heat.

Stage 2
The rice will now begin to fry, so keep stirring it. After a minute it will look slightly translucent. Add the vermouth or wine and keep stirring – it will smell fantastic. Any harsh alcohol flavours will evaporate and leave the rice with a tasty essence.

Stage 3
Once the vermouth or wine has cooked into the rice, add the first ladle of hot stock and a good pinch of sea salt. Turn down the heat to a highish simmer so the rice doesn't cook too quickly on the outside. Keep adding ladlefuls of stock, stirring and almost

massaging the creamy starch from the rice, allowing each ladleful to be absorbed before adding the next. This will take around 15 minutes. Taste the rice – is it cooked?

Carry on adding stock until the rice is soft but with a slight bite. Don't forget to check the seasoning carefully and add salt and black pepper if necessary.

Stage 4
Remove from the heat and add the butter and Parmesan. Stir gently. Place a lid on the pan and allow to sit for 2 to 3 minutes. This is the most important part of making the risotto, as this is when it becomes outrageously creamy and oozy like it should be. Eat as soon as possible while the risotto retains its perfect texture.

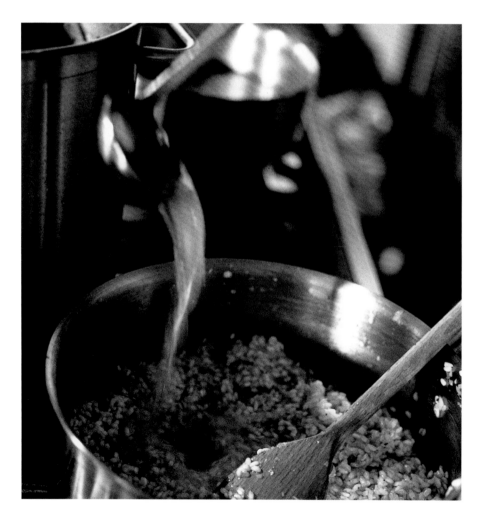

CALORIES	FAT	SAT FAT	PROTEIN	CARBS	SUGAR	SALT	FIBRE
521kcal	18g	9.9g	15.4g	64g	6g	0.8g	2.3g

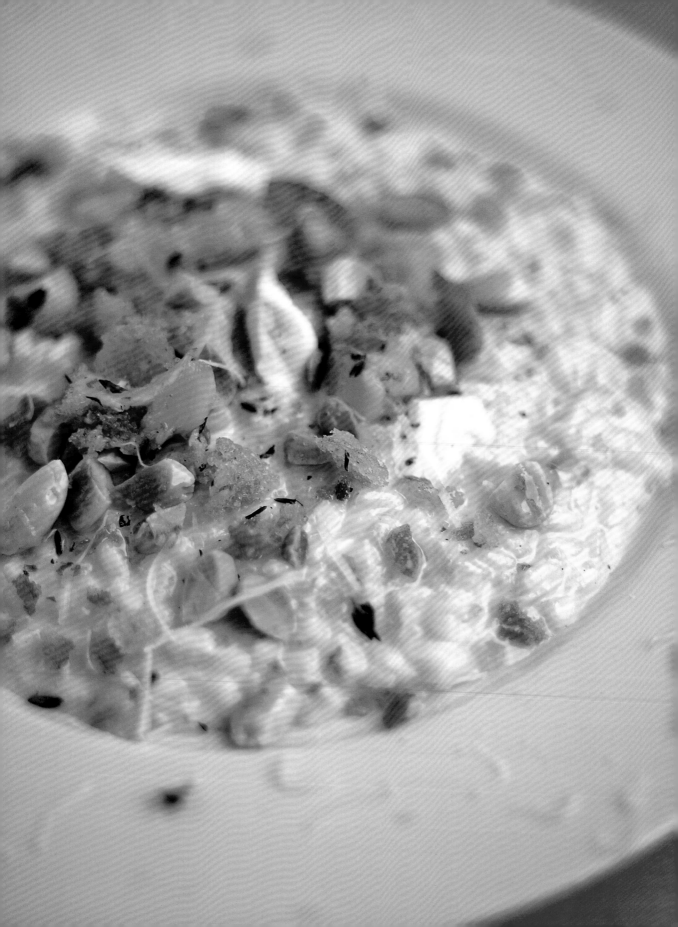

roasted sweet garlic, thyme & mascarpone risotto with toasted almonds & breadcrumbs

Don't be scared by this one – the garlic is not overpowering, it's an extremely subtle and delicate combination.

serves 6

1 × basic risotto recipe (see pages 134–5)
2 large bulbs of garlic, whole and unpeeled
1 good handful of fresh thyme, leaves picked
150g blanched almonds, lightly crushed, cracked or chopped
2 handfuls of coarse fresh breadcrumbs
olive oil
2 heaped tablespoons mascarpone cheese

Roast the whole garlic bulbs in the oven at 230°C/450°F/gas 8 for about 30 minutes, or until soft. Separate the cloves and squeeze out the sweet insides. Add with the thyme leaves at the start of Stage 3 of the basic risotto recipe. In a frying pan, toast the almonds and breadcrumbs in a little oil until crisp and golden. Season with a little sea salt. Set to one side. Serve the risotto with a dollop of mascarpone on the top and sprinkle over the toasted almonds and breadcrumbs. Lovely.

CALORIES	FAT	SAT FAT	PROTEIN	CARBS	SUGAR	SALT	FIBRE
781kcal	39.6g	15.6g	23.6g	73.1g	8.2g	1.1g	2.7g

white risotto with lemon thyme, sliced prosciutto, pecorino & crumbled goat's cheese

I initially made this risotto pretty much off the cuff with leftover cheese from my fridge and a snip of lemon thyme from my window box. It was perfect. Use normal thyme if you can't get hold of lemon thyme.

serves 6
1 × basic risotto recipe (see pages 134–5)
2 good handfuls of fresh lemon thyme, leaves picked
100g pecorino cheese
8 slices of prosciutto
150g goat's cheese

At the start of Stage 3 of the basic risotto recipe add the lemon thyme leaves. When you stir in the butter and Parmesan at Stage 4, grate in the pecorino. Lay over the prosciutto slices just before eating and serve with the goat's cheese crumbled over the top. Scatter with a few extra thyme leaves, if you like.

CALORIES	FAT	SAT FAT	PROTEIN	CARBS	SUGAR	SALT	FIBRE
701kcal	32.4g	18.6g	27.7g	64.8g	6.3g	2.6g	2.7g

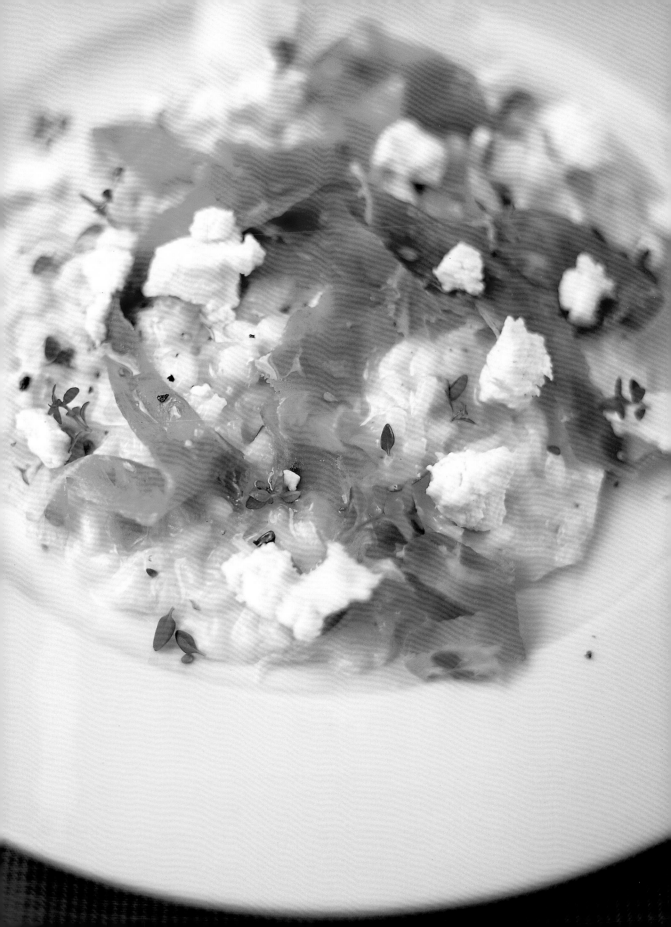

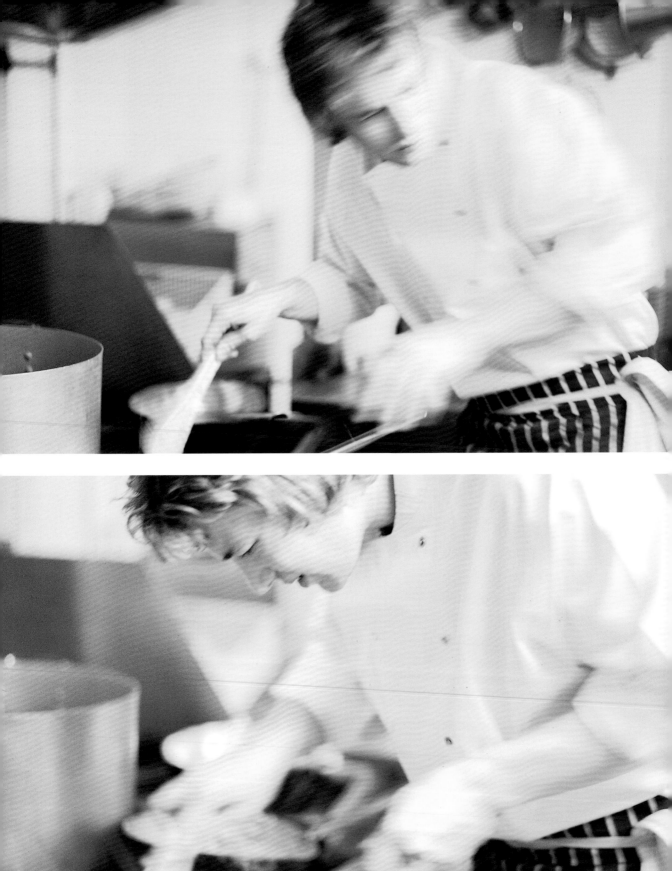

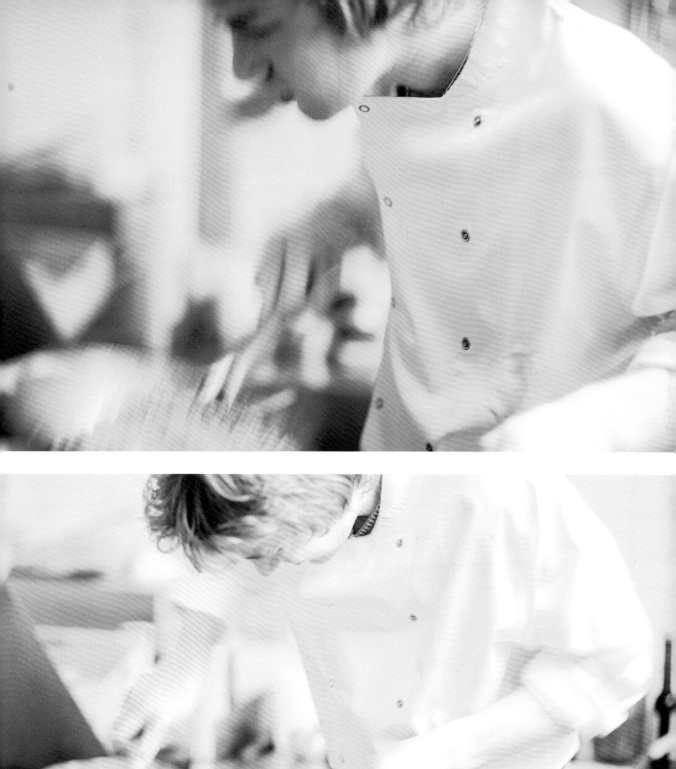

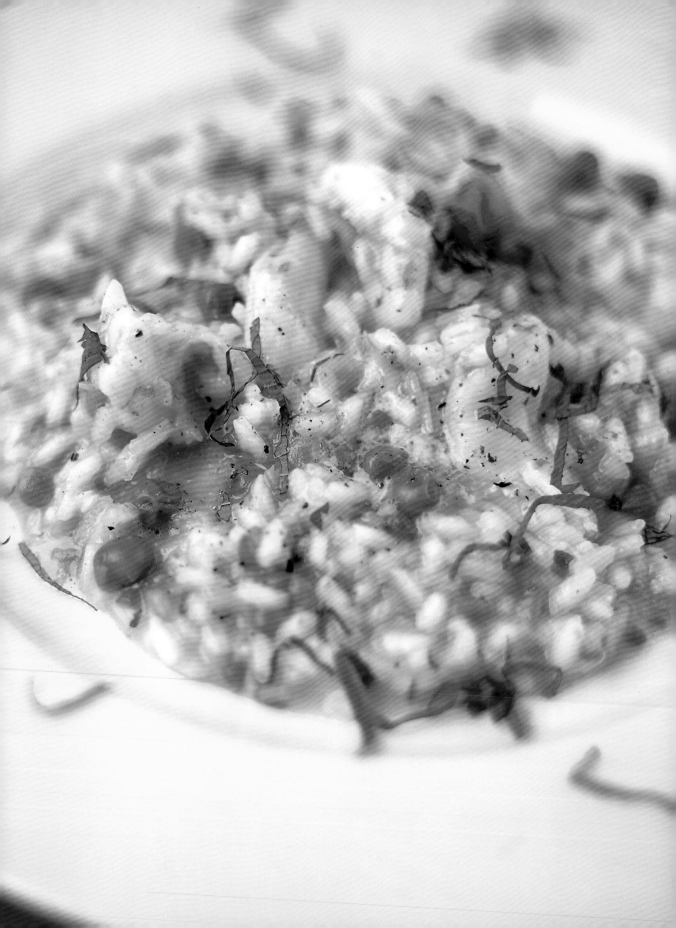

prawn & pea risotto with basil & mint

For me this risotto really works because of the natural sweetness you get in peas and prawns. With a little help from some delicate herbs it will put a smile on your face. Remember not to use any Parmesan in your basic risotto recipe – not so good with fish. If using fresh peas, add the pods to the stock to give it a good pea flavour rather than throw them away. Results with good frozen peas are also brilliant.

serves 6
1 × basic risotto recipe (see pages 134–5), minus the Parmesan cheese
3 good handfuls of fresh peas, podded
1 knob of unsalted butter
450g raw peeled prawns
1 handful of fresh basil, leaves picked and chopped
½ a handful of fresh mint, leaves picked and chopped
1 lemon
extra virgin olive oil

Fry half the peas in the butter and a little stock. Cook until tender and mash. Add this at the end of Stage 3 of the basic risotto recipe with the prawns and the rest of the peas and simmer for 2 minutes – prawns and peas take no time to cook. At Stage 4 throw in the fresh herbs and squeeze in the lemon juice. Stir and serve immediately, drizzled with really nice peppery extra virgin olive oil.

CALORIES	FAT	SAT FAT	PROTEIN	CARBS	SUGAR	SALT	FIBRE
627kcal	22.6g	12g	29.8g	65.9g	6.4g	1.2g	3g

risotto of radicchio, smoky bacon, rosemary & red wine

serves 6

1 × basic risotto recipe (see pages 134–5), minus the vermouth or
   white wine
3 wine glasses of your favourite full-bodied red wine
10 rashers of smoked streaky bacon, finely sliced
olive oil
2 heads of radicchio, trimmed and finely sliced
1 handful of fresh rosemary, leaves picked
1 small knob of unsalted butter

Add the red wine in place of the vermouth or white wine at Stage 2 of the basic
risotto recipe. Fry your bacon in a little oil until slightly golden. Add the radicchio and
rosemary leaves to the pan with the butter and cook gently with the lid on until wilted.
At the start of Stage 3, stir in the bacon, radicchio and rosemary.

CALORIES	FAT	SAT FAT	PROTEIN	CARBS	SUGAR	SALT	FIBRE
593kcal	23.7g	12.1g	18.6g	63.6g	5.4g	1.3g	3.5g

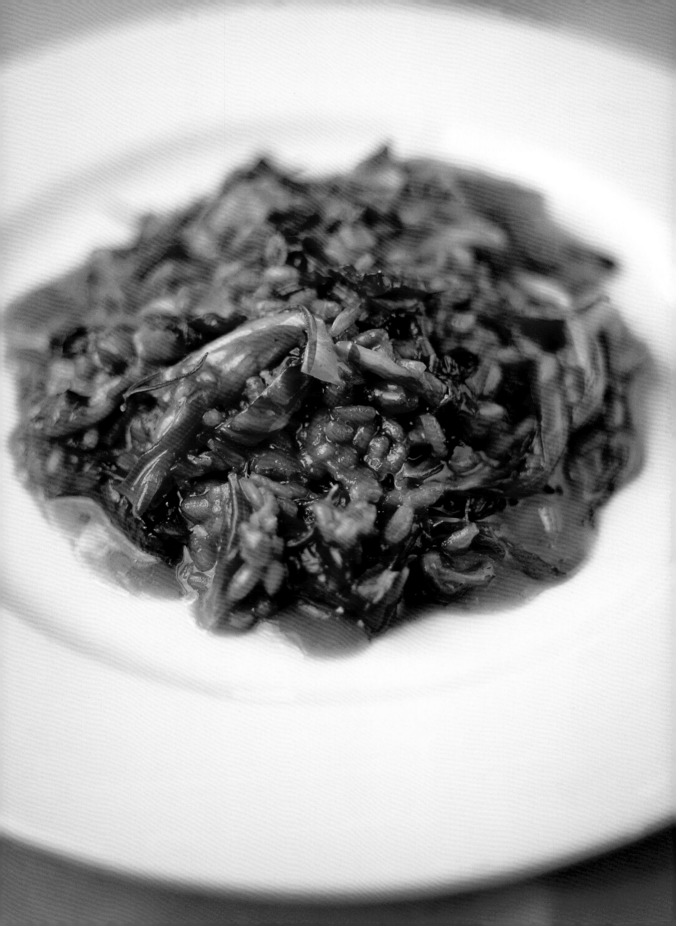

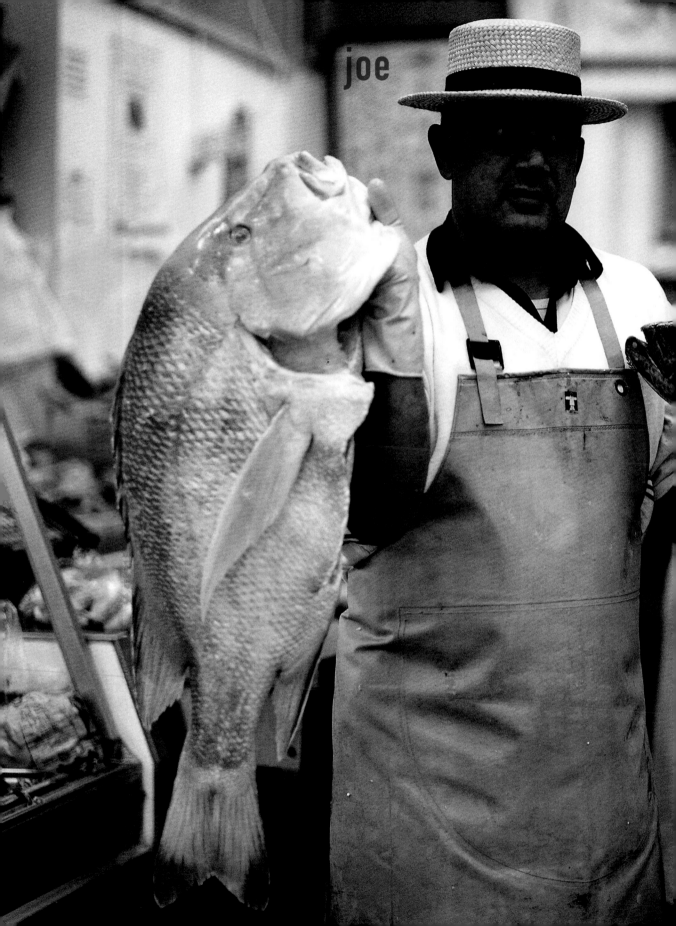

joe

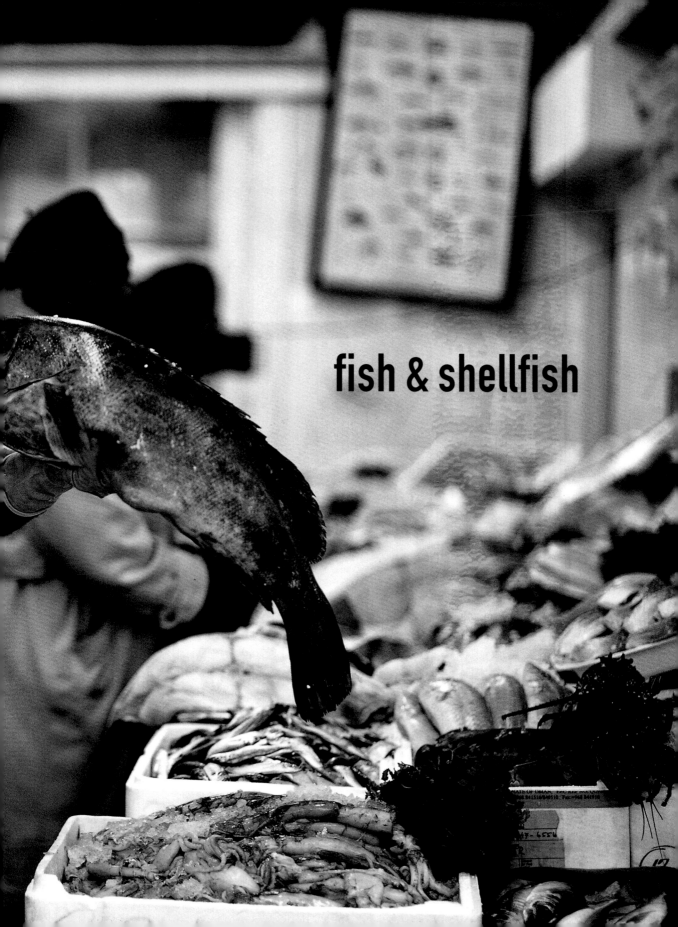

fish & shellfish

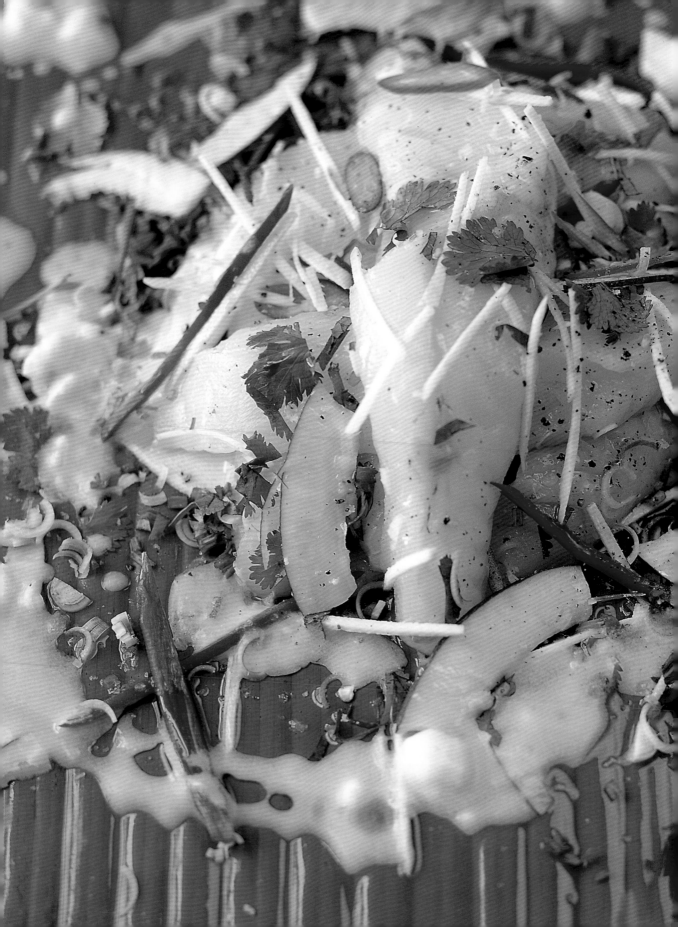

monkfish wrapped in banana leaves
with ginger, coriander, chilli & coconut milk

You can't go wrong with this combination of flavours. It's open to all white fish, especially swordfish, cod, haddock and monkfish. Banana leaves are very easy to buy from oriental stores – get nice big ones to wrap your fish up in. Failing banana leaves, you can use vine leaves which you can get in the supermarkets – somewhat smaller, but no less tasty. If you really can't get hold of any leaves, tin foil will do.

serves 4

4 large banana leaves or vine leaves

olive oil

2 limes

2 fresh red or green chillies

2 sticks of lemongrass, outer leaves removed, finely chopped

1 clove of garlic, peeled and finely chopped

2 good handfuls of fresh coriander, roughly chopped

2 tablespoons sesame seed oil

10cm piece of fresh ginger, peeled and finely sliced

4 × 150g monkfish fillets

1 × 400ml tin of light coconut milk

4 fresh rosemary sprigs, to secure

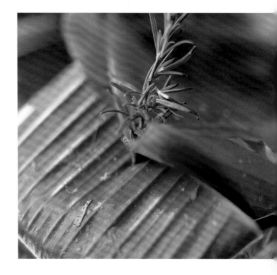

Preheat the oven to 230°C/450°F/gas 8. Lay out the banana leaves and rub them with a little olive oil. Grate over half the lime zest and squeeze over half the juice. Leaving aside the fish, coconut milk and rosemary sprigs, sprinkle a little bit of everything else on one end of each leaf. Place the fish on top, then sprinkle what's left over them, including the remaining lime zest and juice. Pour 5 to 6 tablespoons of coconut milk over each before folding the leaf over the fish, bringing the sides in and spiking it with a rosemary sprig to secure. This will look lovely and it's natural, but I have been known to use a clothes peg or string to hold it all together. It won't be a perfect seal but this allows it to breathe and steam, letting the flavours infuse. Put the parcels on a tray and bake for 15 minutes, then remove from the oven and allow to rest for 5 minutes.

I serve the individual parcels on plates at the table and let my friends dissect them. When opened, the fragrant steam wafts up and smells fantastic. Serve with fluffy rice to mop up the juices – that's all it has to be. End of story, done, lovely.

fish & shellfish

CALORIES	FAT	SAT FAT	PROTEIN	CARBS	SUGAR	SALT	FIBRE
255kcal	14.8g	6.5g	25.1g	5.4g	3.1g	0.1g	0.9g

traybaked cod with runner beans, pancetta & pine nuts

Another superb combination. The runner beans, pancetta and pine nuts go amazingly well together. It's a great way to cook the cod because it's all in one tray, which means hardly any washing up.

serves 4
700g runner beans, trimmed and sliced at an angle
1 clove of garlic, peeled and finely sliced
olive oil
4 × 225g cod steaks, on the bone
12 rashers of pancetta or smoked dry-cured streaky bacon, thinly sliced
1 good handful of pine nuts
2 lemons, halved

Preheat the oven to 220°C/425°F/gas 7. Place the runner beans in a roasting tray. Throw in the garlic and a little sea salt and black pepper, add 2 tablespoons of oil, and mix it all around to coat. Nestle the cod steaks in among the runner beans, lightly season again, then place the pancetta over the cod and among the beans. Sprinkle with pine nuts and drizzle a little oil over the top. Take the lemon halves and place them in the tray – they will cook and colour slightly, going jammy, sweet and lemony.

Cook for 15 minutes in the middle of the oven. Lightly lay tin foil over the fish for the first 5 minutes, then remove it. You know the cod is cooked when the bone in the middle is easily removed. This is a meal in itself, so serve with all the lovely juices from the tray drizzled over the top.

CALORIES	FAT	SAT FAT	PROTEIN	CARBS	SUGAR	SALT	FIBRE
420kcal	18.9g	3.4g	55.3g	7.4g	5.6g	1.4g	6g

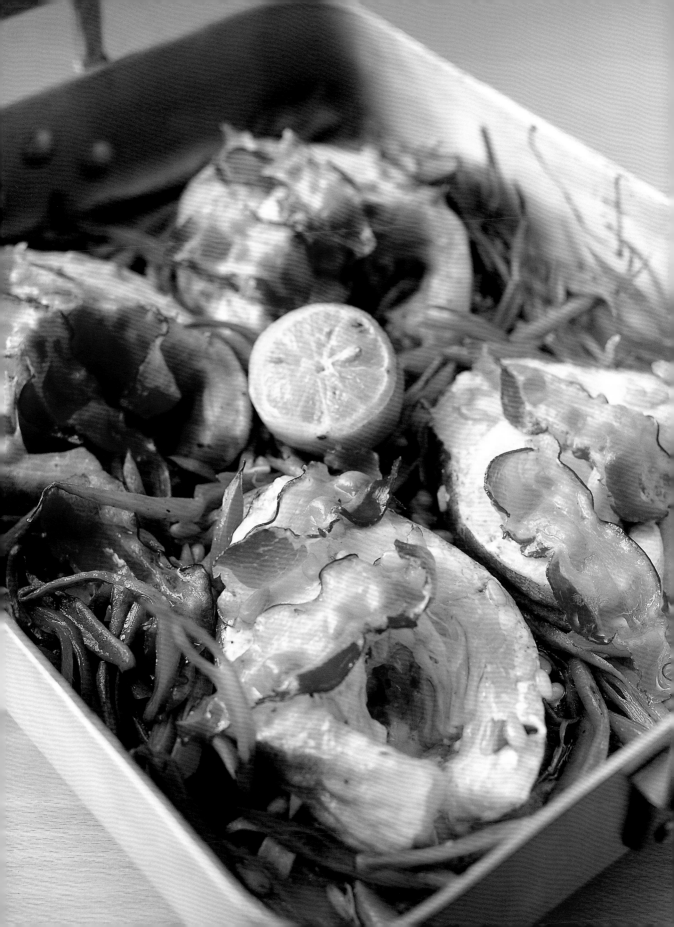

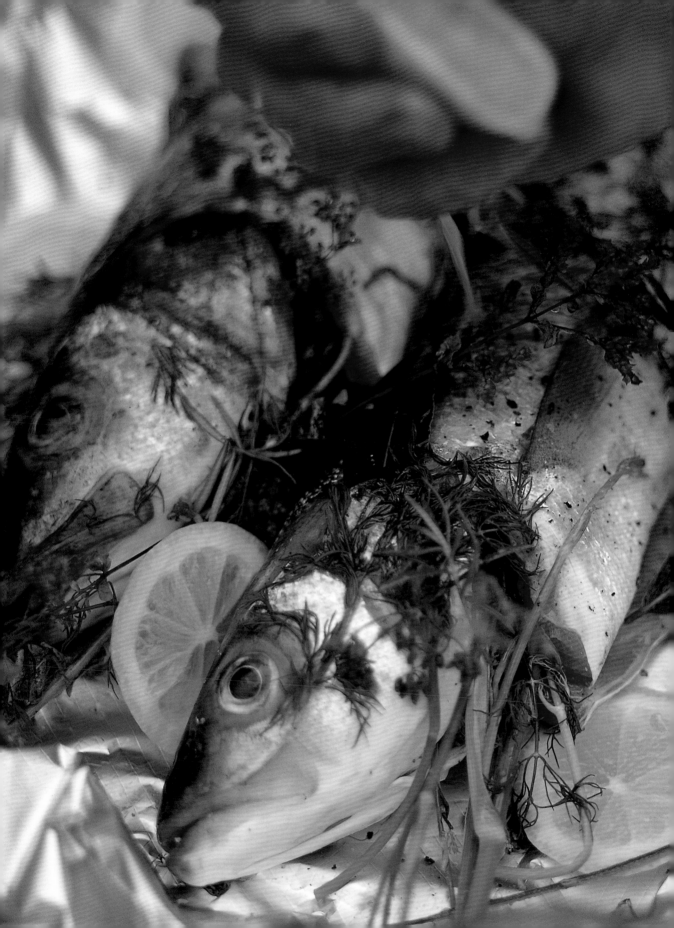

whole sea bass baked in a bag & stuffed with herbs

This is a great way to cook fish, letting it retain all its natural juices and rewarding you with the most fantastic tasty sauce. I think the fish is best served in its bag in the middle of the table – it's real theatre. When the bag is broken open the fragrant smells waft all around the table, leaving everyone salivating for it.

serves 4

1 × 1.8kg sea bass or 2 × 900g sea bass, scaled and gutted
1 red onion, peeled and finely sliced
1 bulb of fennel, finely sliced
1 clove of garlic, peeled and finely chopped
1 dessertspoon fennel seeds
4 handfuls of mixed fresh herbs, such as flat-leaf parsley, basil,
    fennel, dill, tarragon, marjoram, bay
3 lemons
6 good lugs of olive oil

Preheat the oven to 220°C/425°F/gas 7. Tear off a piece of tin foil 5 times as long as the fish, then fold this in half to give you double thickness. In the middle of one half of the foil sprinkle the red onion, fennel and garlic. Place the fish snugly on top of the veg. Season the inside and outside of the fish with sea salt, freshly ground black pepper and the fennel seeds, then stuff with all the herbs – use just one herb or a mixture of your favourites. Squeeze over the juice of 2 of the lemons, slice the third lemon and tuck around the fish, and pour over the oil.

Fold the foil over the fish and seal the three edges neatly and tightly, being careful not to pierce the foil as this will let the juices escape. Cook in the preheated oven for 10 minutes per 450g. Allow the fish to rest for 5 minutes before serving at the table. Nice with simple boiled potatoes and a crisp salad.

fish & shellfish

153

CALORIES	FAT	SAT FAT	PROTEIN	CARBS	SUGAR	SALT	FIBRE
853kcal	57.7g	11.2g	79.2g	5.1g	4.2g	1.3g	0.6g

wok-cooked fragrant mussels

I had the idea for this dish while eating mussels in New York. It takes literally minutes to cook and tastes absolutely pukka. Simply serve with plain boiled or steamed rice.

serves 4–6
2kg mussels, scrubbed, debearded
olive oil
2 cloves of garlic, peeled and finely sliced
3 sticks of lemongrass, outer leaves removed, finely sliced
2 fresh red or green chillies
10cm piece of fresh ginger, peeled and finely sliced
2 handfuls of fresh coriander, pounded or finely chopped
1 tablespoon sesame seed oil
5 spring onions, trimmed and finely sliced
3 limes
1 × 400ml tin of light coconut milk

Place the mussels and a couple of lugs of olive oil in a large, very hot wok or pot. Shake around and add the rest of the ingredients, apart from the limes and coconut milk. Keep turning over until all the mussels have opened – throw away any that remain closed. Squeeze in the lime juice and add the coconut milk, then season to taste with sea salt and black pepper. Bring to the boil and serve immediately.

fish & shellfish

CALORIES	FAT	SAT FAT	PROTEIN	CARBS	SUGAR	SALT	FIBRE
311kcal	18.5g	7.1g	24.4g	11.3g	3.7g	1.3g	0.8g

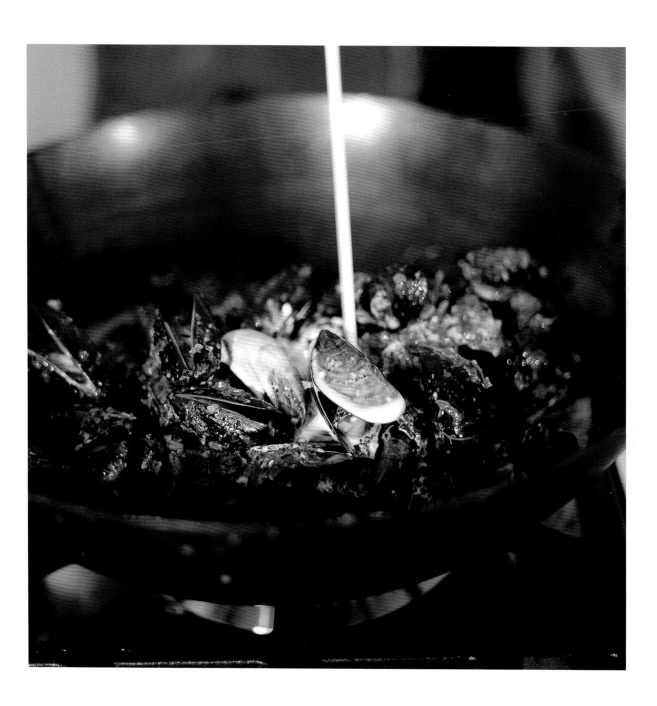

roasted fillet of sea bass stuffed with herbs, baked on mushroom potatoes with salsa verde – à la Tony Blair

I cooked this for Tony Blair and the Italian prime minister at the British/Italian summit. It went down a treat so I thought I'd put it in the book. This is a really great way to cook sea bass. Try to get the fattest bass fillets you can find. Failing that, royal bream is fantastic cooked this way, too.

serves 4
4 × 225g sea bass fillets
1 handful of mixed fresh herbs, such as green or purple basil,
    flat-leaf parsley, thyme, roughly chopped
1kg potatoes, scrubbed
olive oil
2 cloves of garlic, peeled and finely chopped
3 knobs of unsalted butter
450g mixed, preferably wild, mushrooms, torn
3 lemons
4 tablespoons salsa verde (see page 277)

Preheat the oven to 240°C/475°F/gas 9. Put a bit of greaseproof paper on the bottom of a baking tray, rubbed with oil. Slash the fish fillets about halfway down and stuff the slashes with the herbs. Slice the potatoes lengthways, just under 1cm thick. Dry them with kitchen paper and very lightly coat with oil. Mix in half the garlic, season with sea salt and black pepper, then lay them out in one layer on the tray. Cook the potatoes in the oven for around 15 minutes, or until just cooked. Remove and put to one side.

Put the rest of the garlic into a pan with 2 good knobs of butter and a lug of oil. Fry the mushrooms and season – if water comes out of them, just continue cooking until it evaporates. Take the pan off the heat, squeeze in the juice from 1 lemon and stir in the remaining knob of butter. Scatter the mushrooms over the potatoes and kind of rub them in on top, underneath, all over. Place the sea bass fillets on top. Now bake in the oven for 12 to 15 minutes, depending on the thickness of the fish.

Remove the tray from the oven, cover with tin foil and leave to sit for 5 minutes, during which time all the lovely juices will run out into the potatoes. Serve each portion with 1 tablespoon of salsa verde, half a lemon and a glass of crisp white wine.

CALORIES	FAT	SAT FAT	PROTEIN	CARBS	SUGAR	SALT	FIBRE
802kcal	45.1g	14.2g	52g	50.2g	2.8g	1.8g	5.4g

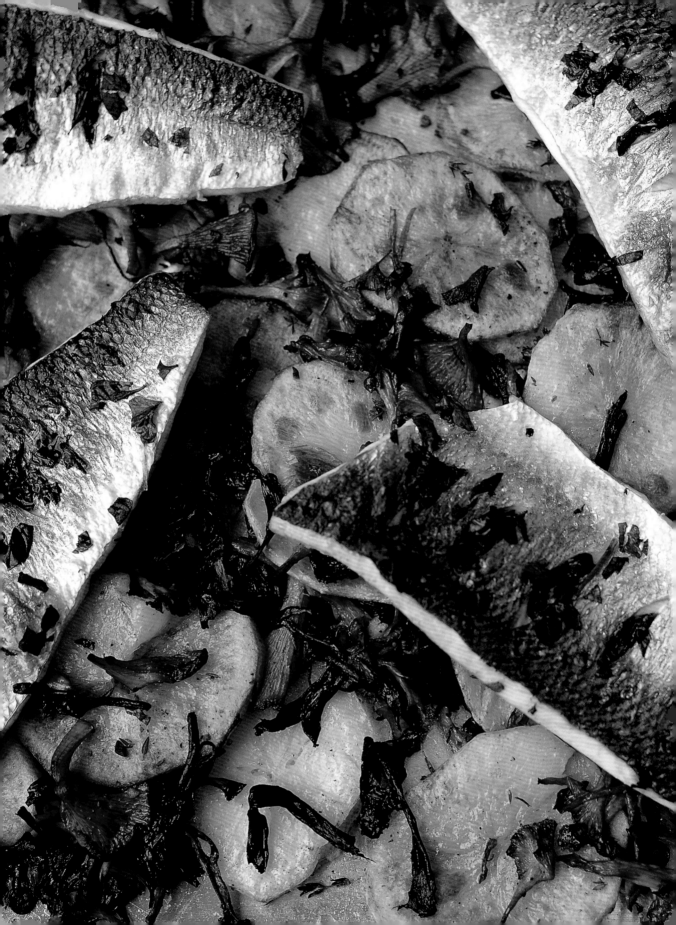

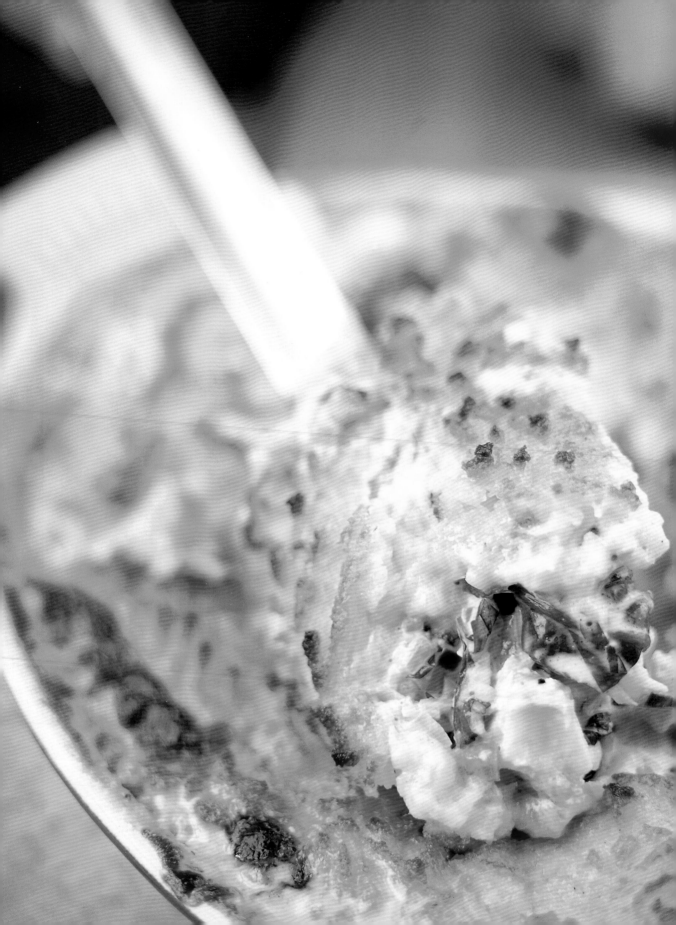

fantastic fish pie

The whole fish pie thing is one of the most homely, comforting and moreish dinners I can think of. This is a cracking recipe which does it for me.

serves 6
5 large potatoes, peeled and diced into 2.5cm chunks
2 large eggs
2 large handfuls of baby spinach
1 onion, peeled and finely chopped
1 carrot, peeled, halved and finely chopped
olive oil
250ml double cream
2 good handfuls of grated mature Cheddar or Parmesan cheese
1 lemon
1 heaped teaspoon English mustard
1 large handful of fresh flat-leaf parsley, finely chopped
450g haddock or cod fillet, skin off, pin-boned and sliced into strips
optional: 1 whole nutmeg, for grating

Preheat the oven to 230°C/450°F/gas 8. Put the potatoes into boiling salted water and bring back to the boil for 2 minutes. Carefully add the eggs to the pan and cook for a further 8 minutes, or until hard-boiled, by which time the potatoes should also be cooked. At the same time, steam the spinach in a colander above the pan. This will only take a minute. When the spinach is done, remove from the colander and gently squeeze out any excess moisture. Drain the potatoes in the colander. Remove the eggs, cool under cold water, then peel and quarter them. Place to one side.

In a separate pan, slowly fry the onion and carrot in a little oil for about 5 minutes, then add the double cream and bring just to the boil. Remove from the heat and add the cheese, lemon juice, mustard and parsley. Put the spinach, fish and eggs into an earthenware dish and mix together, pouring over the creamy vegetable sauce. The cooked potatoes should be drained and mashed – add a bit of oil, sea salt, black pepper and a touch of nutmeg (if using). Spread on top of the fish. Don't bother piping it to make it look pretty – it's a homely hearty thing. Place in the oven for 25 to 30 minutes, or until the potatoes are golden. Serve with some nice peas or greens, not forgetting your baked beans and tomato ketchup. Tacky but tasty, and that's what I like.

CALORIES	FAT	SAT FAT	PROTEIN	CARBS	SUGAR	SALT	FIBRE
539kcal	30.4g	18.3g	23.3g	45.7g	6.1g	0.6g	5.4g

seared scallops & crispy prosciutto
with roasted tomatoes & smashed white beans

serves 4

4 large ripe plum tomatoes, quartered

1 pinch of dried oregano

olive oil

8 slices of prosciutto

1 small clove of garlic, peeled and finely chopped

1–2 small dried red chillies, crumbled to taste

4–6 anchovy fillets, in oil, chopped

1 × 400g tin of cannellini beans or flageolet beans, drained

extra virgin olive oil

12 scallops, trimmed, with roe on or off to your preference

1 × extra virgin olive oil & lemon juice dressing (see page 81)

1 small handful of peppery leaves, such as rocket or watercress

Preheat the oven to full whack (240°C/475°F/gas 9). Season the tomatoes and sprinkle with the oregano. Drizzle with olive oil and roast in the oven skin side down for about 10 to 15 minutes. Place the prosciutto slices beside the tomatoes and continue to roast for a further 10 minutes, or until the tomatoes are juicy and the prosciutto is crisp. In a pan, fry the garlic, chillies and anchovies in a lug of olive oil for a minute or so. Add the beans and cook for a couple of minutes before adding a wineglass of water. Bring to the boil, then lightly mash to a coarse purée. Loosen the purée with a little more water, if needed. Finish with some peppery extra virgin olive oil, sea salt and black pepper.

Season the scallops, then sear in a frying pan with a touch of olive oil for 2 minutes without touching them. Check and continue to fry until they have a lovely sweet caramelized outside – turn them over and allow the other side to do the same. Don't overcook them. Remove to a bowl and coat with 1 tablespoon of extra virgin olive oil & lemon juice dressing. Put some smashed bean purée on each plate, scatter over the tomatoes, prosciutto and scallops, and finish off with some peppery leaves.

CALORIES	FAT	SAT FAT	PROTEIN	CARBS	SUGAR	SALT	FIBRE
411kcal	16.3g	2.8g	42.3g	22g	3g	3.3g	6.8g

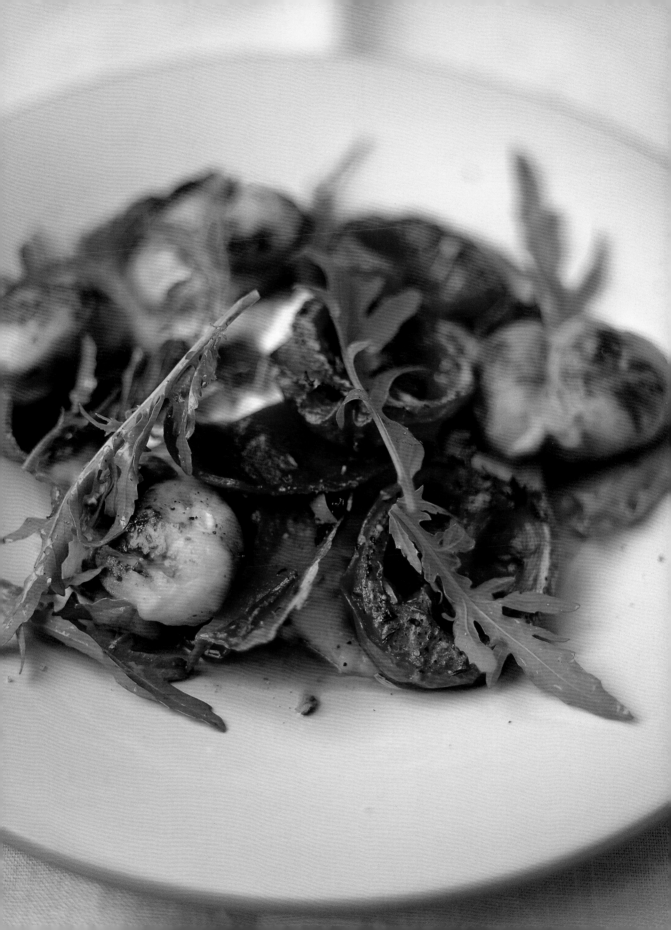

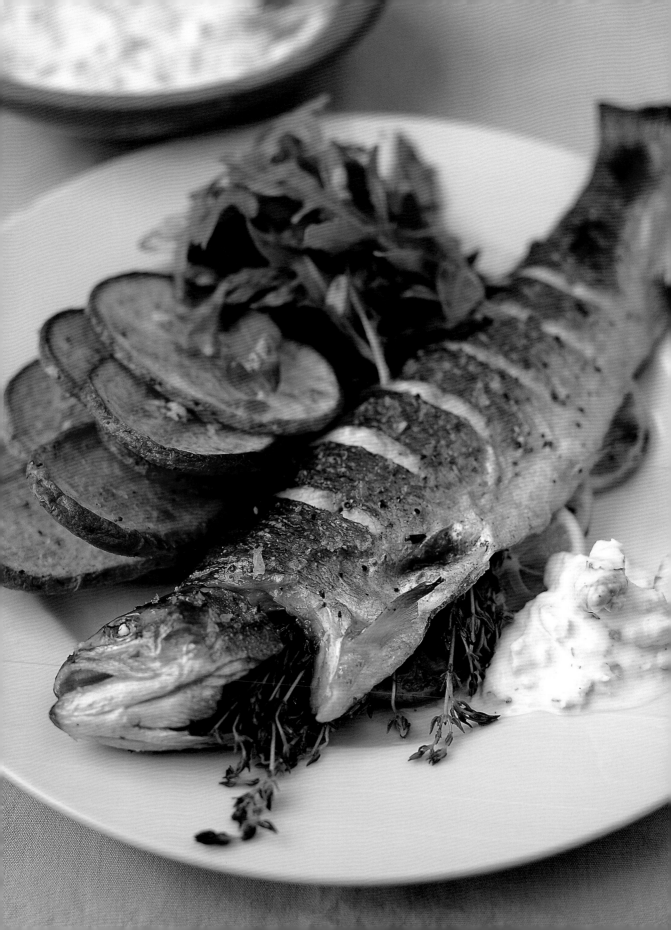

baked trout & potatoes
with a crème fraîche, walnut & horseradish sauce

Trout is a fantastic and readily available fish. The combination of hot horseradish, nutty walnuts and creamy crème fraîche is a pukka marriage with trout as well as with the more obvious beef and lamb.

serves 4
450g potatoes, peeled and finely sliced
olive oil
4 × 400g whole trout, scaled and gutted
1 heaped tablespoon freshly grated horseradish
250g crème fraîche
2 handfuls of fresh walnuts, shelled and crushed
1 lemon

optional
a little fresh thyme
1 lemon, sliced

Preheat the oven to full whack (240°C/475°F/gas 9). Dry the sliced potatoes with kitchen paper and lightly coat with oil. Season with sea salt and black pepper and place in a single layer in a large roasting tray. Place on a low oven shelf and roast for 15 minutes, or until golden and crisp. Meanwhile, pat the trout dry, then with a sharp knife slash each fish at an angle on both sides – this will allow the heat and seasoning to penetrate. Rub with oil and a pinch of salt and pepper. For extra flavour you can stuff the fish with fragrant herbs. I like to use thyme with some lemon slices, too. This should only take a couple of minutes. Cook for around 12 minutes at the top of the oven until crisp and golden.

While the fish and potatoes are cooking, make the sauce. Fresh horseradish, which you should peel and grate, is nicer, but you can also use the creamed horseradish bought in jars. Not quite as hot but still tasty. Mix the horseradish in a bowl with the crème fraîche and walnuts, then season to taste with salt, pepper and lemon juice.

Serve the fish and potatoes side by side with a good lob of the crème fraîche sauce. Really nice with a green salad, some buttered bread and a glass of beer.

CALORIES	FAT	SAT FAT	PROTEIN	CARBS	SUGAR	SALT	FIBRE
744kcal	48.9g	18.4g	53.5g	24.3g	2.9g	2.2g	2.7g

grilled swordfish, green beans & spicy tomato salsa

serves 4

4 × 175g swordfish steaks, ideally 1cm thick
olive oil
5 handfuls of mixed salad leaves, such as watercress, rocket,
    radicchio, chicory, dandelion
2 handfuls of green beans
1 × extra virgin olive oil & lemon juice dressing (see page 81)
1 × tomato salsa recipe (see page 277)

Rub the swordfish steaks with a little oil, sea salt and black pepper. Place on a very hot griddle pan or barbecue and char for 2 minutes on each side. Remove from the pan. Cook the beans in boiling salted water until tender, then drain. Lightly dress the beans and salad leaves with the extra virgin olive oil & lemon juice dressing. Rip up the swordfish and place it in and among the beans and salad leaves. Spread over the spicy tomato salsa before serving.

CALORIES	FAT	SAT FAT	PROTEIN	CARBS	SUGAR	SALT	FIBRE
509kcal	37.7g	6g	35.3g	7.4g	6.3g	1.8g	3.4g

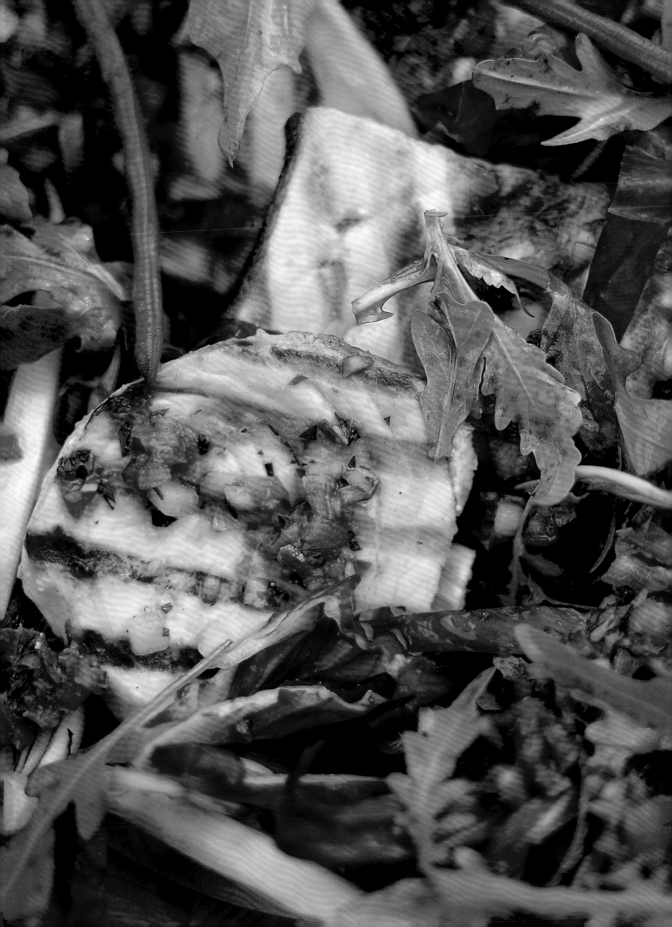

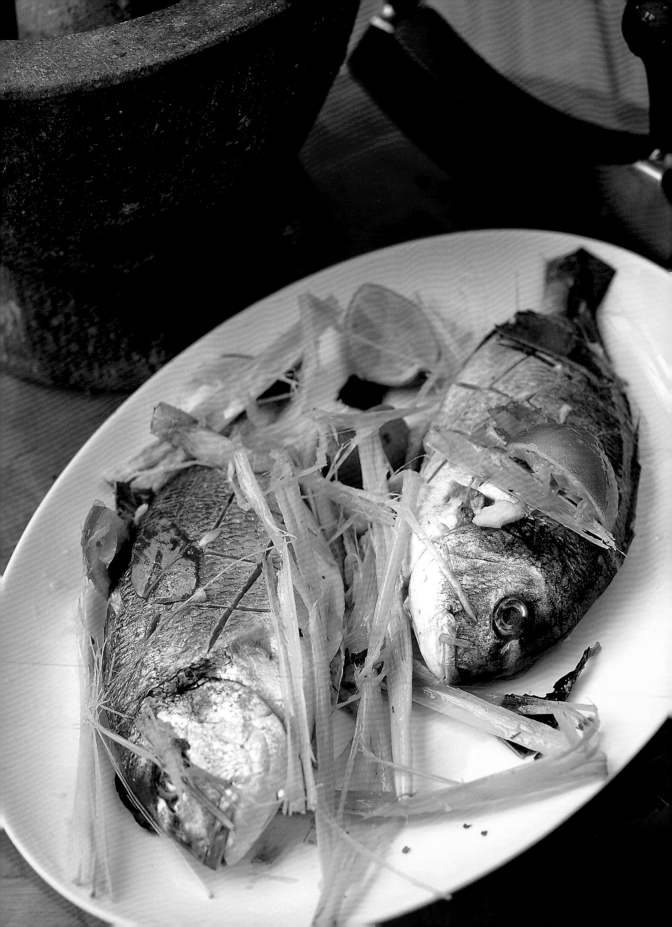

wok-fried crispy bream
with steamed greens & Thai dressing

serves 2
2 × 300g royal or grey bream, scaled and gutted
1 × Asian marinade (see page 194)
sunflower oil
plain flour, for dusting
2 good handfuls of Chinese greens, such as spinach,
    pak choi, bok choi, Chinese broccoli
½ × Thai dressing (see page 80)

Slash the bream on both sides, about 1cm deep, in a criss-cross fashion. In a pestle and mortar, pound up the marinade and rub it all over the fish, getting it into the cuts and the belly. Let this sit in the fridge for up to an hour.

Heat a wok with 5 to 7.5cm of sunflower oil in. Put a bit of potato into the oil and when it is nicely golden you know the wok is hot enough – be very careful with the hot oil. Remove the bream from the marinade and pat dry with kitchen paper. Dust each fish with flour, shaking off any excess, then carefully place each fish in the wok and fry for 3 minutes on each side – the skin will go amazingly crispy. Steam the greens in a colander above boiling water until tender. To serve, place the greens on a plate, put the fish on top, and drizzle with the Thai dressing.

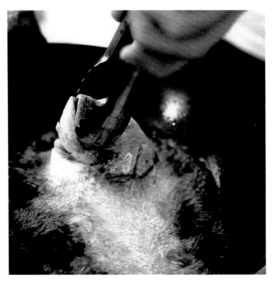

CALORIES	FAT	SAT FAT	PROTEIN	CARBS	SUGAR	SALT	FIBRE
919kcal	75.9g	9.8g	36.4g	23.8g	3.3g	2.2g	1.2g

salmon fillet wrapped in prosciutto
with herby lentils, spinach & yoghurt

serves 4

250g lentils

4 × 225g salmon fillets, skin off

8 slices of prosciutto

olive oil

1 lemon

2 good handfuls of mixed fresh herbs, such as flat-leaf parsley,
    basil, mint, leaves picked and chopped

3 large handfuls of baby spinach, chopped

extra virgin olive oil

4 tablespoons natural yoghurt

Preheat the oven to 220°C/425°F/gas 7. Put the lentils into a pan, cover with water, bring to the boil and simmer until tender. Season the salmon fillets with a little black pepper before wrapping them in the prosciutto slices. Leave some of the flesh exposed. Drizzle with oil and roast in the oven for around 10 minutes, or until the prosciutto is golden. Feel free to cook the salmon for less time if pinker is to your liking. Drain away most of the water from the lentils and season carefully with sea salt, pepper, the lemon juice and 4 good lugs of extra virgin olive oil. Just before serving, stir the herbs and spinach into the lentils on a high heat, until wilted. Place on plates with the salmon and finish with a drizzle of lightly seasoned yoghurt.

CALORIES	FAT	SAT FAT	PROTEIN	CARBS	SUGAR	SALT	FIBRE
946kcal	61.2g	10.9g	68.2g	32.9g	3g	1.9g	6.1g

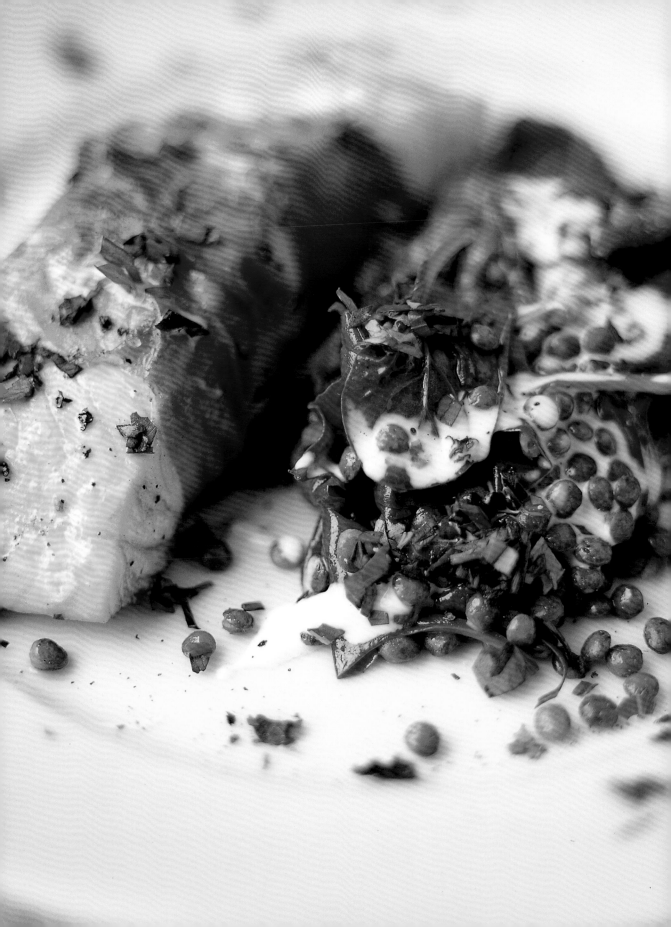

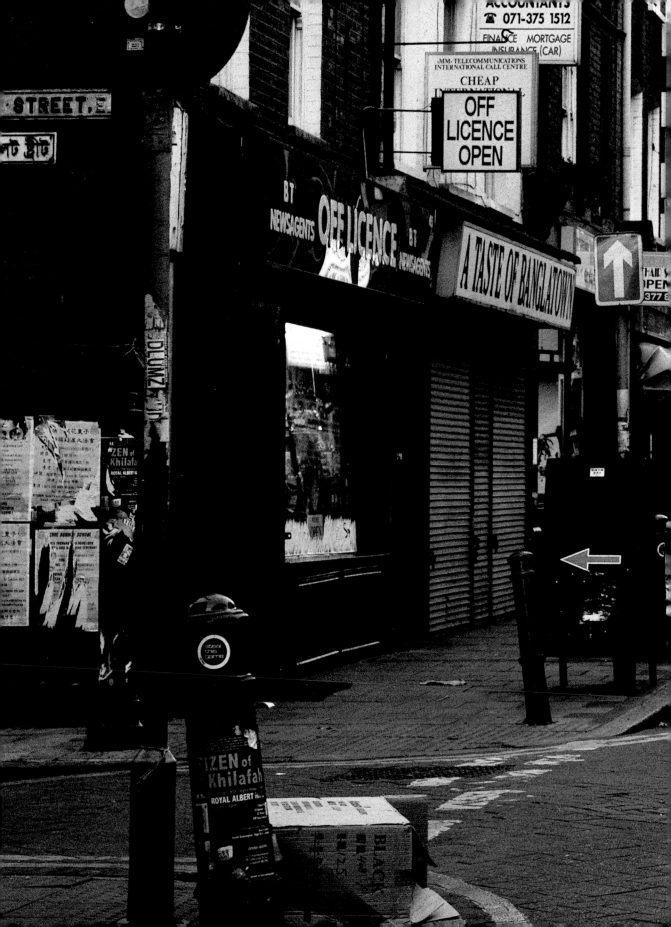

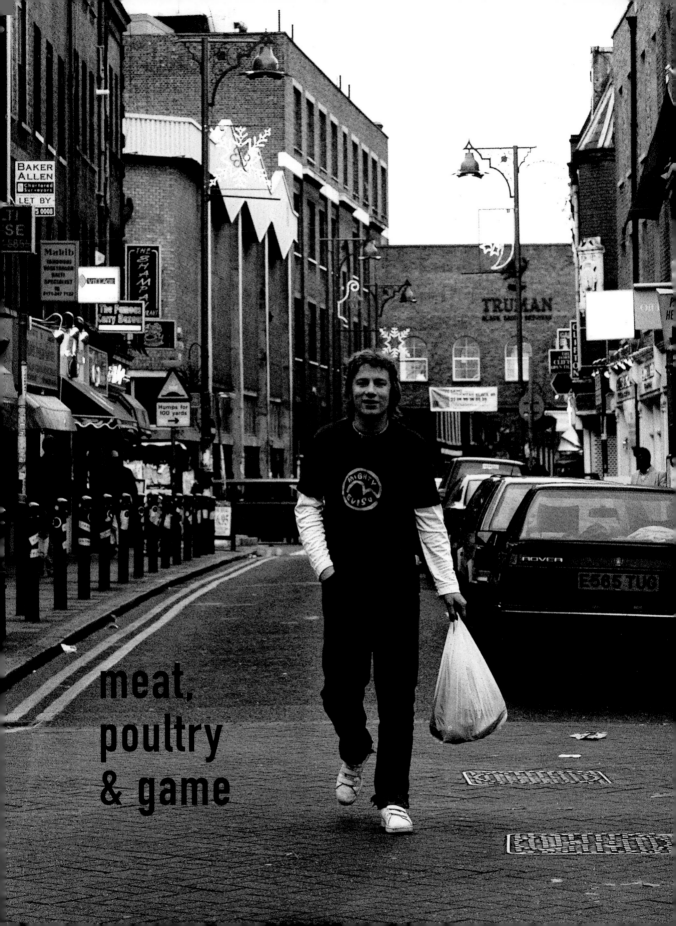

meat,
poultry
& game

roast loin of pork with peaches

Pork, peaches, butter and thyme is one of the most luscious combinations I've ever had. You must try it.

serves 6
1 × six-rib loin of pork
1 bunch of fresh thyme, leaves picked and chopped
80g unsalted butter (at room temperature)
8 fresh peaches (or use 2 tins with natural juice), halved and destoned

Preheat the oven to 220°C/425°F/gas 7. Score the pork skin about 1cm apart through the fat nearly to the meat. With a knife carefully part the meat from the ribs. Scrunch the chopped thyme leaves into the butter with some sea salt and black pepper. Rub and distribute a little of the butter into the gap you have made between the ribs and the meat. Push in as many peaches as you can fit and pack the rest of the butter on top. To hug the meat and ribs together and hold the peaches in place, simply fasten some butcher's string around the pork loin in 3 or 4 places and tie firmly. Place in a roasting tray with any leftover peaches and other veg you wish to cook with it – potatoes, parsnips, celeriac and Jerusalem artichokes are all good – and cook for 50 minutes to 1 hour, allowing it to rest for 10 minutes before serving. I usually make a little bit of homemade gravy in the roasting tray after removing the pork and veg. The sticky, marmitey goodness is great when boiled with a little water or wine and any extra juices from the pork. Tasty.

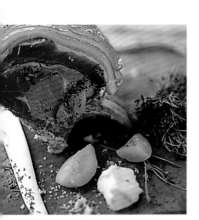 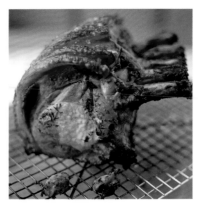 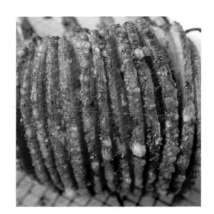

CALORIES	FAT	SAT FAT	PROTEIN	CARBS	SUGAR	SALT	FIBRE
521kcal	42.1g	18.4g	27.9g	7.9g	7.3g	0.7g	0.6g

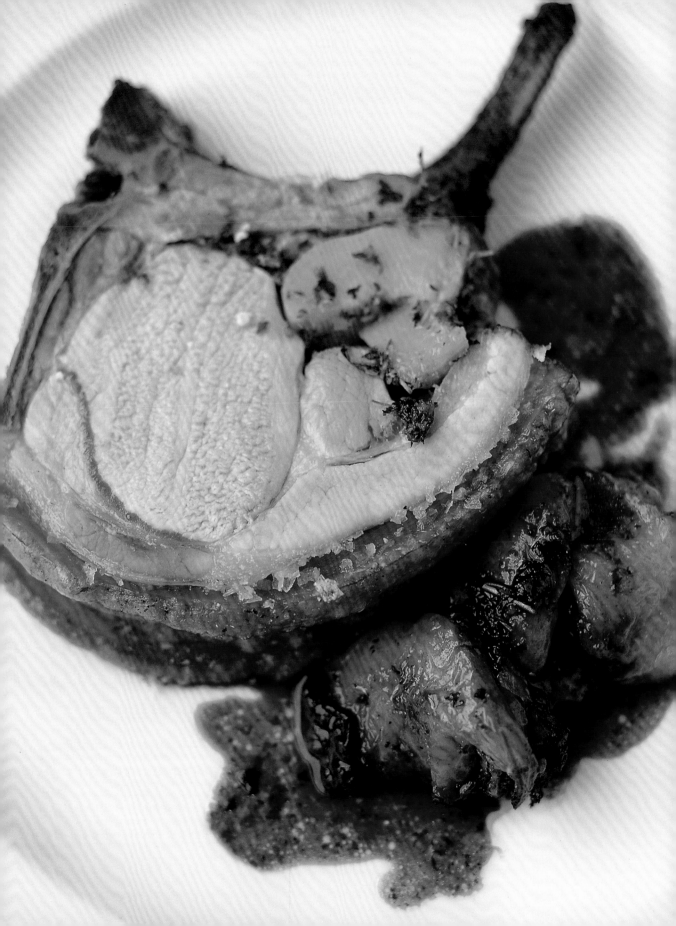

braised five-hour lamb with wine, veg & all that

This is a real hearty and trouble-free dinner. There's barely any preparation, just a nice long cooking time which will reward you with the most tender meat and tasty sauce. Large legs of lamb are ideal for this dish, as they benefit from slow cooking. If using a smaller leg of spring lamb, consider cooking for an hour less.

serves 6
1 x 2kg leg of lamb
olive oil
6 rashers of dry-cured smoked streaky bacon, thickly sliced
3 red onions, peeled and quartered
3 cloves of garlic, peeled and sliced
2 good handfuls of mixed fresh herbs, such as thyme, rosemary, bay
4 large potatoes, peeled and cut into chunks
1 celeriac, peeled and cut into chunks
6 large carrots, scrubbed and halved
3 parsnips, scrubbed and halved
1 bottle of white wine

Preheat the oven to 170°C/325°F/gas 3. Season the lamb with sea salt and black pepper. In a large casserole pot or a deep-sided roasting tray, fry the lamb in a couple of good lugs of oil until brown on all sides. Add the bacon, onions and garlic and continue to fry for 3 more minutes. Throw in the herbs and veg, pour in the wine plus an equivalent amount of water, bring to the boil, and tightly cover with tin foil. Roast for 5 hours, or until tender, seasoning the cooking liquor, to taste. To serve, pull away a nice portion of meat, take a selection of veg and serve with some crusty bread.

CALORIES	FAT	SAT FAT	PROTEIN	CARBS	SUGAR	SALT	FIBRE
679kcal	24.5g	7.8g	35.4g	60.4g	21.4g	0.7g	16.1g

seared carpaccio of beef

The reason I like to make this dish is because, apart from being really quick and simple, it's a sociable feast where everyone can tuck in and help themselves. I love all that. I always serve this on a large plate in the middle of the table, with crusty bread and a glass of wine. Any leftovers are even more gorgeous the next day in a nice firm bap.

A good carpaccio is always made from a prime cut of meat or fish, like fillet or loin, and it's normally served completely rare. To make it different I sear it lightly, adding fantastic flavour to the outside, but still leaving it delicately and classically raw.

Here I will show you how to sear a fillet of beef with a tasty crust, followed by two of my favourite ways of serving it.

serves 6
1 heaped tablespoon coriander seeds
1 handful of fresh rosemary, leaves picked and finely chopped
dried oregano
1.5kg fillet of beef

Pound the coriander seeds in a pestle and mortar, then mix in the rosemary leaves, add a pinch each of sea salt, black pepper and oregano, and sprinkle on to a board. Roll and press the fillet of beef over this, making sure all the mixture sticks to the meat. In a very hot griddle pan, or on a barbecue, sear the meat for around 5 minutes, or until brown and slightly crisp on all sides. Remove from the pan. Allow to rest for 5 minutes, then slice it all up as thinly as you can, laying the slices on a large plate as you go.

meat, poultry & game

CALORIES	FAT	SAT FAT	PROTEIN	CARBS	SUGAR	SALT	FIBRE
352kcal	15.5g	7.1g	53.2g	0.2g	0g	0.6g	0.7g

seared carpaccio of beef with roasted baby beets, creamed horseradish, watercress & Parmesan

serves 6–8

700g baby beetroot

olive oil

10 tablespoons balsamic vinegar

1.5kg fillet of beef

100g freshly grated or creamed horseradish

200g crème fraîche

1 splash of white wine vinegar

1 lemon

3 good handfuls of watercress

extra virgin olive oil

100g freshly shaved Parmesan cheese

Preheat the oven to 230°C/450°F/gas 8. Wash and scrub the beets, trim the ends, and toss into a roasting tray with a little olive oil, the balsamic vinegar and a pinch of sea salt and black pepper. Cover with tin foil and roast until tender. Cooking time depends on size.

After preparing the beef (see page 175), sprinkle the roasted beetroots randomly (whole, halved or quartered, depending on size) over the sliced meat. Now mix the horseradish and crème fraîche together, tweaking with vinegar and lemon juice, to taste. Drizzle this over the beetroot. Dress some watercress with extra virgin olive oil and lemon juice. Scatter this, along with some small shavings of Parmesan, all over the plate and get ready to tuck in!

CALORIES	FAT	SAT FAT	PROTEIN	CARBS	SUGAR	SALT	FIBRE
519kcal	21.5g	10.4g	62.8g	19.4g	17.7g	1.5g	4.1g

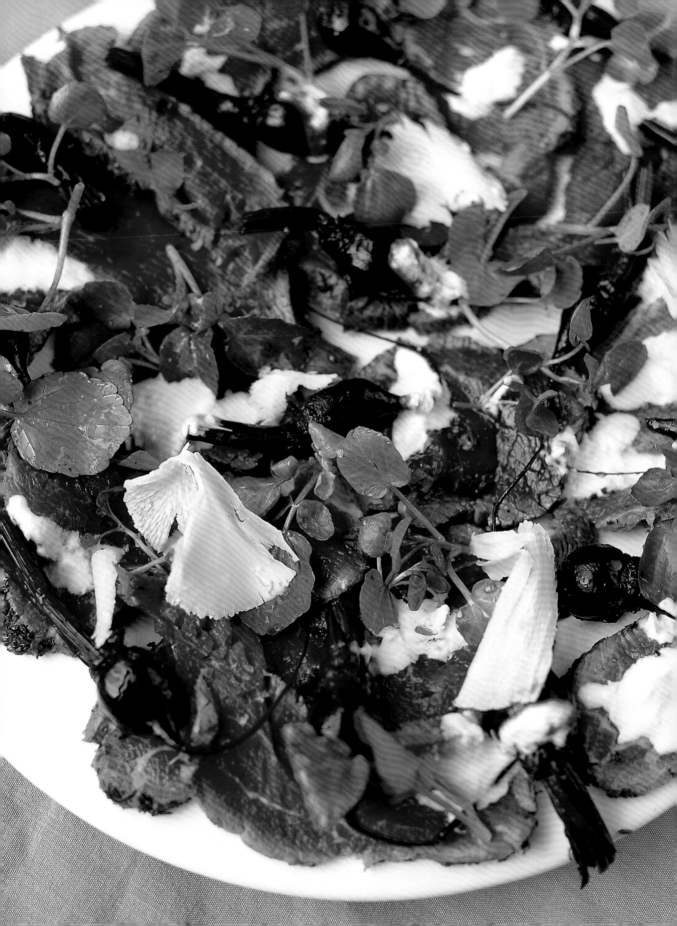

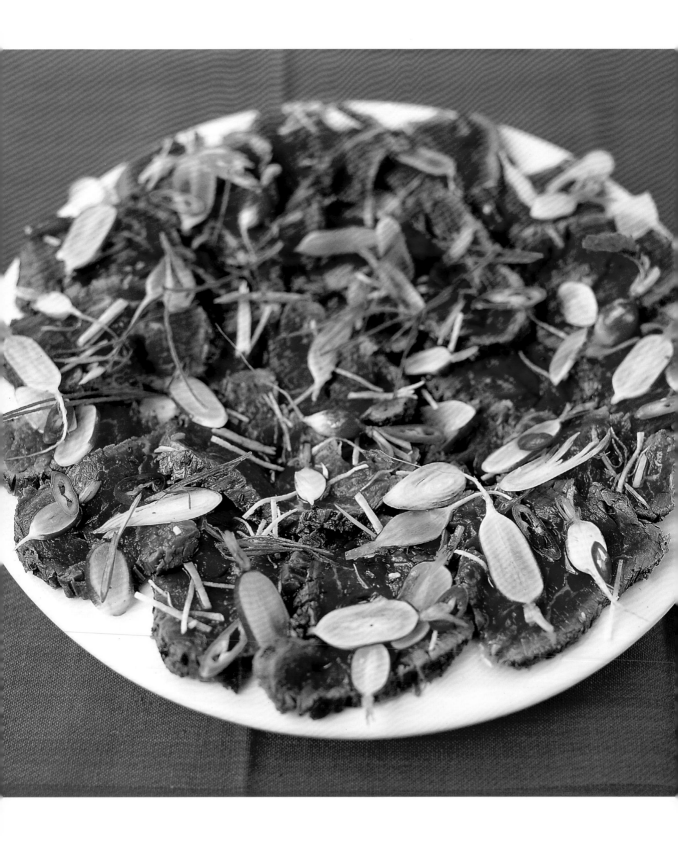

seared carpaccio of beef with chilli, ginger, radish & soy

This is really good served with crunchy Thai salad (see page 67) and crusty bread.

serves 6–8
1.5kg fillet of beef
5cm piece of young, fresh ginger, peeled and very finely sliced
2–3 fresh red or green chillies, deseeded and finely sliced
1 good handful of radishes, finely sliced
1 small handful of fresh coriander stalks, finely sliced lengthways
sesame seed oil
low-salt soy sauce
2 limes

After preparing the beef (see page 175), gather the ginger slices and cut finely across into little delicate matchsticks. Flick these randomly over the beef with the chillies, radishes and coriander. Drizzle with a very small amount of sesame seed oil and some soy sauce, then squeeze over the lime juice, making sure each slice of meat gets an equal dousing, and tuck in!

CALORIES	FAT	SAT FAT	PROTEIN	CARBS	SUGAR	SALT	FIBRE
369kcal	16.8g	7.2g	53.7g	1.3g	0.7g	0.8g	0.9g

traybaked pork chops with herby potatoes, parsnips, pears & minted bread sauce

When I make this dish I ask my butcher to slice me a two-rib pork chop. I then ask him to lose one of the ribs and a little of the fat and to bat the meat out slightly, leaving me with a huge pork chop that looks fantastic.

serves 4
8 pork chops, or 4 double pork chops
½ × rosemary, garlic & lemon marinade (see page 194)
3 parsnips
3 smooth-skinned pears
700g potatoes, scrubbed
1 × minted bread sauce recipe (see page 278)

Rub and massage the pork chops with the rosemary marinade and, ideally, leave for 1 to 6 hours for maximum flavour. Preheat the oven to 220°C/425°F/gas 7. Wash the parsnips and pears and slice into quarters lengthways, removing the cores from the pears, then cut the potatoes into ½cm thick pieces. Dry with kitchen paper, then put them into a roasting tray with the parsnips, pears, pork chops and the marinade. Toss to lightly coat everything, then season with sea salt and black pepper and roast in the oven for 45 minutes to an hour, depending on the size of the chops.

While the chops and veg are cooking, make the minted bread sauce. It's great spread all over the pork.

CALORIES	FAT	SAT FAT	PROTEIN	CARBS	SUGAR	SALT	FIBRE
989kcal	64.5g	19.1g	44.2g	61.6g	17.6g	1.1g	11.5g

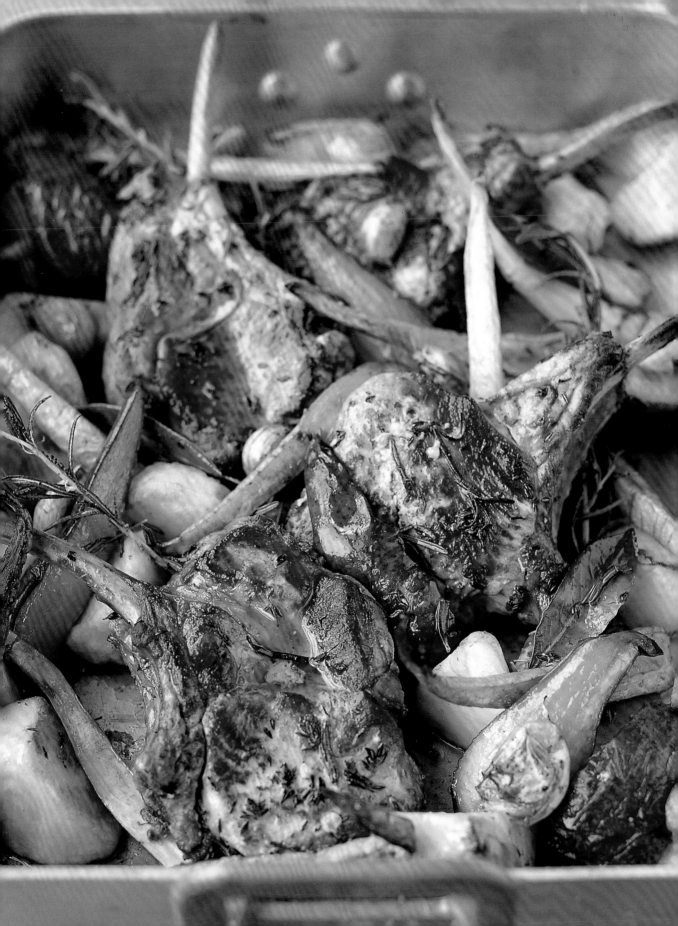

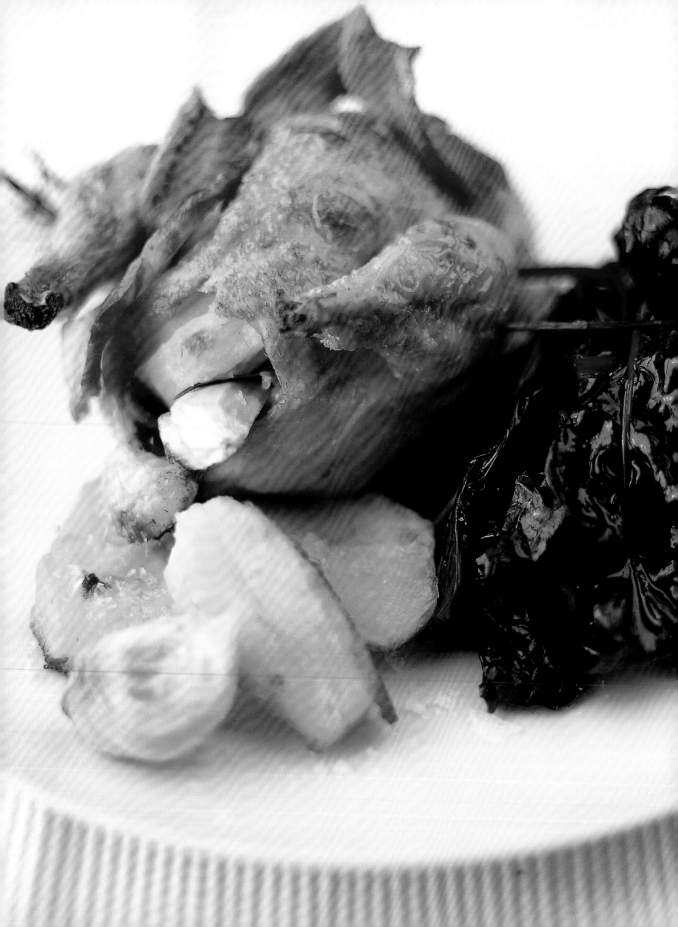

roasted Hamilton poussin wrapped
with streaky bacon & stuffed with potatoes and sage

This is nothing to do with the Duke of Hamilton. It's a scrumptious recipe that my handsome art director Johnny Boy Hamilton cooks for his lovely wife. Lucky woman. There is something quite cute about the individual chicken thing, and cooking the potatoes in the cavities seems to make them taste even better.

serves 4

450g potatoes, peeled and quartered

4 poussin chickens

1 handful of fresh sage, thyme or rosemary

olive oil

12 cloves of garlic

12 rashers of dry-cured smoked streaky bacon, thinly sliced

1 glass of white wine

optional: double cream

Preheat the oven and a roasting tray to 220°C/425°F/gas 7. Boil the potatoes in boiling salted water until nearly cooked. Drain and allow to cool, then put into a bowl. Remove any fat from inside each chicken cavity. Season the potatoes with sea salt and black pepper, add the freshly torn herbs and enough oil just to coat, and toss. Stuff the chickens with half the potatoes and herbs. Put them into the hot roasting tray with the garlic and the rest of the potatoes and roast for 30 minutes. After this time the chicken should be looking as handsome as its inventor and the skin should be crisp and golden. At this point lay the streaky bacon snugly over the breast meat. Cook for another 15 minutes.

Remove the chickens from the oven, take them out of the tray and rest for 5 minutes while you make a quick bit of gravy. I normally remove as much fat as possible from the tray before placing it on the hob on a gentle heat. Splash a glass of white wine into it, then boil up and scrape away all the goodness from the sides of the tray. Simmer for a couple of minutes. It's not a thick, robust gravy, just a tasty gesture. (A nice option at this point is to add a little cream to the gravy, which works really well.) Served with something nice and green like steamed spinach or chard, and the potatoes pulled out from inside the chickens, it all goes down a treat. Nice one, John.

CALORIES	FAT	SAT FAT	PROTEIN	CARBS	SUGAR	SALT	FIBRE
802kcal	49.6g	13.1g	57.6g	25.1g	1.5g	1.9g	2.4g

fantastic roasted chicken

This roasted chicken is really tasty. The principle is very similar to the perfect roast chicken recipe in my first book, getting fantastic flavours right into the bird.

serves 6
1.8kg chicken
1 large lemon
8 slices of prosciutto or Parma ham, thinly sliced
1–2 cloves of garlic, peeled and finely chopped
2 good handfuls of fresh thyme, leaves picked and finely chopped
100g unsalted butter (at room temperature)
1kg potatoes, peeled and cut into chunks
1 large celeriac, peeled

Preheat the oven and a roasting tray to 220°C/425°F/gas 7. Using your fingers, part the chicken breast skin from the breast meat. It's important to try to push your hand gently down the breast, being careful not to rip the skin. With a speed-peeler, remove the fragrant yellow rind of the lemon, keeping the peeled lemon to one side. Tear up the prosciutto and place in a bowl with the lemon rind, garlic and thyme. Season with sea salt and black pepper, then scrunch it all into the butter. Push this into the space you have made between the meat and the skin – rub and massage any that's left over in and around the bird. It's all tasty stuff. I could tell you to tie the chicken up but I've decided it's a palaver and not worth it in this case. Slash the thigh meat to allow the heat to penetrate a little more, which makes it taste better. Cut the peeled lemon in half and push it into the cavity, then put the chicken into the hot roasting tray and roast for 25 minutes.

   While the chicken is cooking, parboil the potatoes in boiling salted water for 10 minutes, then drain. Cut the celeriac into irregular chunks around the same size as the potatoes. Remove the chicken from the oven, by which time the tasty butter will have melted, flavoured and cooked out of the chicken into the bottom of the tray, awaiting your potatoes and celeriac. Normally I put a fork into the cavity of the chicken and lift it out of the tray for 20 seconds while I toss and coat the vegetables in the butter. Put the chicken back on top and cook for 45 minutes. Leave to stand for 10 minutes. Once the meat and vegetables have been removed, a little light gravy can be made in the tray on the hob with a splash of wine and stock, a little simmering and scraping.

CALORIES	FAT	SAT FAT	PROTEIN	CARBS	SUGAR	SALT	FIBRE
706kcal	43.6g	16.9g	44.9g	35.6g	3.5g	1.6g	6.5g

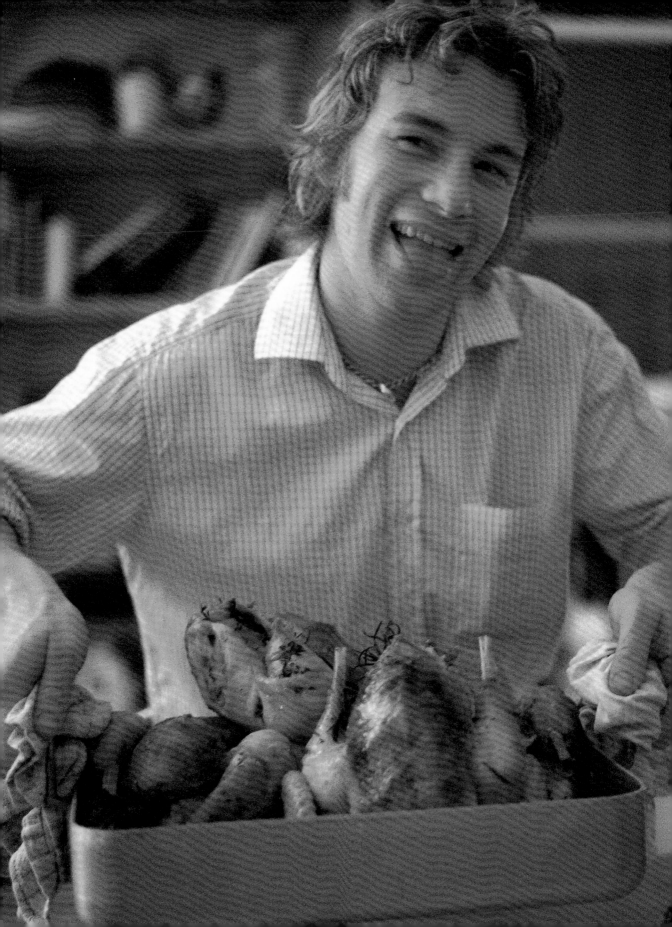

roasted fillet of beef rolled in herbs
& porcini mushrooms & wrapped in prosciutto

As far as roasted meat goes, this is extremely fast and simple, yet decadently rich. One of the tricks, whether you buy it in a deli or a supermarket, is to ask them to slice your prosciutto and lay it side by side on an A3 (ish) sized piece of waxed paper.

serves 4

12 slices of prosciutto or Parma ham
3 cloves of garlic, peeled
1 good handful of dried porcini mushrooms, soaked in 300ml boiling water
3 good knobs of unsalted butter
½ a lemon
1kg centre fillet of beef, trimmed
1 good handful of fresh rosemary and thyme, leaves picked and chopped
2 glasses of red wine

Preheat the oven and a roasting tray to 230°C/450°F/gas 8. Make sure there are no gaps in between the laid-out slices of prosciutto. Drain the porcini mushrooms, reserving the soaking liquor. Chop one of the garlic cloves and fry with the porcini mushrooms in 1 knob of butter for a minute, then add half the soaking liquor (make sure it's grit-free). Simmer slowly and reduce for around 5 minutes before stirring in a squeeze of lemon juice, the remaining 2 knobs of butter and a pinch of sea salt and black pepper. Rub the tasty mushrooms over half the laid-out prosciutto. Season the fillet of beef and roll it in the herbs. Place it on the mushroomy end of the prosciutto and slowly roll up. Once rolled, pull off the paper and push in the ends of the prosciutto to neaten. Lightly secure with 4 pieces of string. Chefs have a certain way of doing this, but as long as the string holds the meat together I don't care how you do it.

Place the fillet in the hot roasting tray with a couple more cloves of garlic and cook for 25 minutes (rare), 30 to 35 minutes (medium), 40 minutes (well-done) or 50 minutes (cremated!). Halfway through, add the wine to the tray. When the meat is done, remove it to a chopping board and leave it to rest for 5 minutes. Pour any juices back into the roasting tray. Simmer the juices on the hob, scraping all the goodness from the sides of the tray. Remove from the heat and serve as a light red wine gravy. Slice the fillet as thick or as thin as you like and serve with some potatoes or gorgeous greens. I like to reserve a little of the cooked porcini to serve with my greens.

CALORIES	FAT	SAT FAT	PROTEIN	CARBS	SUGAR	SALT	FIBRE
630kcal	33.3g	16.4g	63g	3.9g	0.8g	2.8g	1.6g

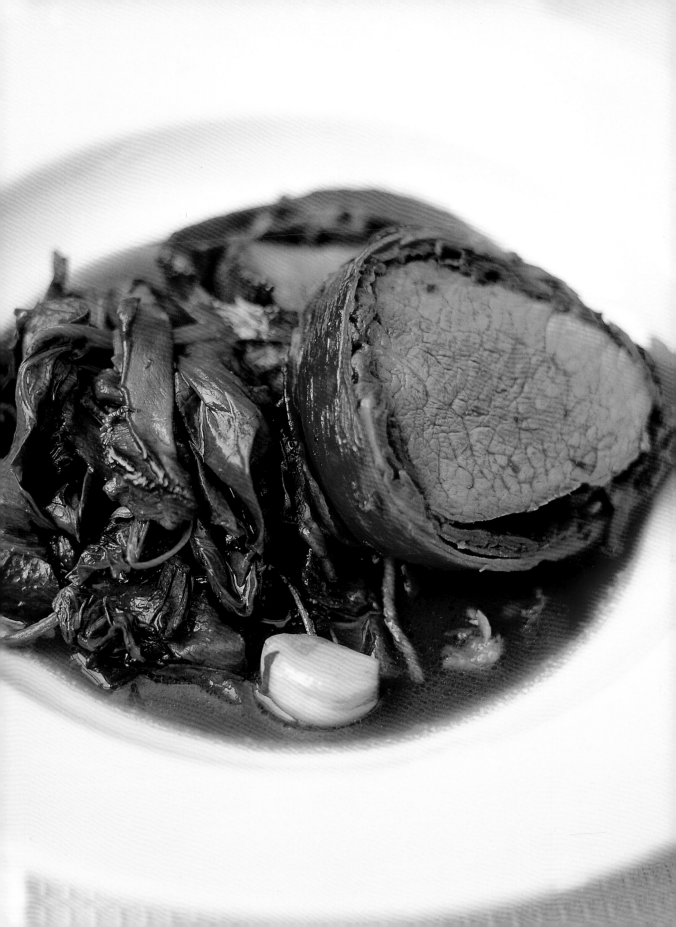

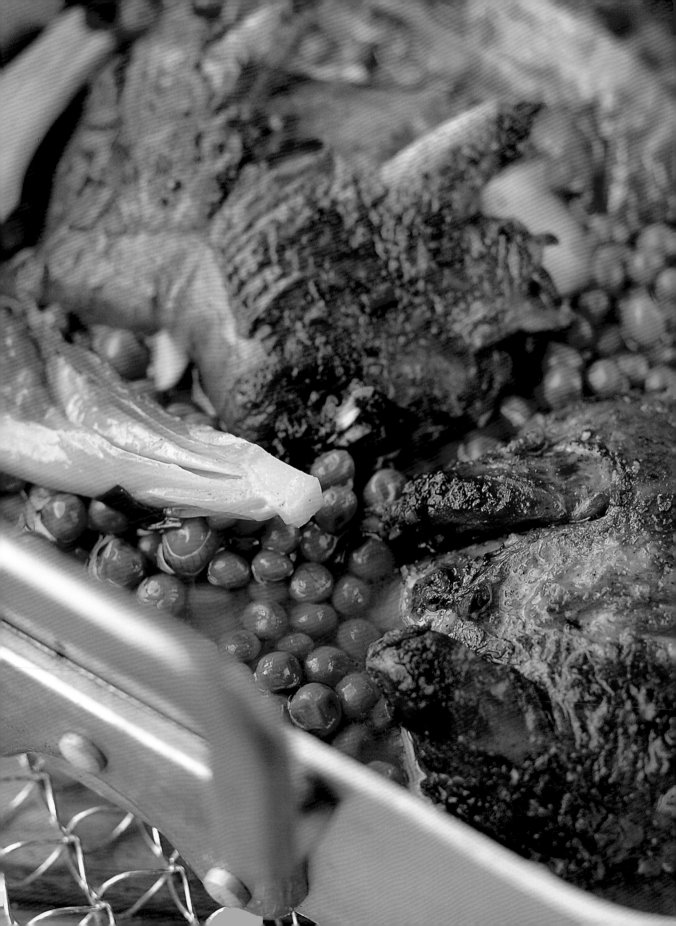

braised pigeon breasts with peas, lettuce & spring onions

You can use whole pigeons in this recipe, but I prefer to remove the bottom of each carcass with a knife or a pair of scissors to open and flatten them out like a book. The cooking time I have given is sufficient, but if you like your meat pink, lessen it.

serves 4
4 pigeons
olive oil
1 bunch of spring onions, stalks chopped and bulbs left whole
1 clove of garlic, peeled and finely chopped
3 good knobs of unsalted butter
1 heaped tablespoon plain flour
1kg peas, fresh or frozen
2 cos lettuces, quartered
1 litre chicken or vegetable stock (see pages 275–6)

Preheat the oven to 220°C/425°F/gas 7 and get a high-sided casserole pan or roasting tray hot on the hob. Prepare the pigeons (see intro), season with sea salt and black pepper, then fry skin side down in the hot pan with a little oil until lightly golden. Remove from the pan and fry the chopped spring onion stalks and garlic for 1 minute, or until slightly softened. Add the butter and flour. Turn the heat down and cook for a further 3 minutes without colouring. Add the peas, spring onion bulbs, lettuce and enough stock to cover, then place the pigeons on top, skin side up. Cook for 20 minutes, then remove from the oven and allow to sit for 5 minutes before serving.

CALORIES	FAT	SAT FAT	PROTEIN	CARBS	SUGAR	SALT	FIBRE
534kcal	23.7g	9.7g	46.2g	36.6g	7.8g	1g	14.9g

Peter's lamb curry

My mate Peter Begg, lovely bloke, fine chef, thoroughbred Scotsman, kilt and no undies, makes the best curry and likes a cold beer. Say no more . . . love him.

serves 8

1 × hot & fragrant rub (see page 195)
2 tablespoons unsalted butter
2 × 400g tins of quality plum tomatoes
300ml stock
1.5kg leg of lamb, bone out, diced
olive oil
1 handful of fresh mint and coriander,
  chopped
250g natural yoghurt
1–2 limes

curry paste

5cm piece of fresh ginger, peeled
2 red onions, peeled
10 cloves of garlic, peeled
2 fresh red chillies
1 bunch of fresh coriander

Preheat the oven to 170°C/325°F/gas 3. Chop the paste ingredients roughly, add the hot & fragrant rub and whiz in a food processor. In a large casserole pan, fry the curry paste in the butter until golden, stirring regularly. Add the tomatoes and pour in the stock (or use water). Bring to the boil, cover with tin foil and place in the oven for 1 hour 30 minutes to intensify the flavours. Remove the foil and continue to simmer on the stove until it thickens – this is your basic curry sauce.

Fry the lamb in a little oil until golden, then add to the curry sauce and simmer for around 1 hour, or until tender. Feel free to vary the curry by using diced chicken, prawns or paneer (see below), or vegetables like Swiss chard, spinach, peas, cauliflower, fried aubergine, okra, boiled potatoes, chickpeas or lentils. Sprinkle with chopped coriander and mint and stir in the yoghurt. Season to taste with sea salt and black pepper and add a good squeeze of lime juice. Serve with spiced breads, steamed basmati rice and lots and lots of cold beer!

CALORIES	FAT	SAT FAT	PROTEIN	CARBS	SUGAR	SALT	FIBRE
450kcal	28.1g	12.7g	41.3g	10.8g	9.1g	0.7g	2.7g

paneer Indian cheese

In a thick-bottomed pan, bring 2 litres of full cream milk to the boil, remove from the heat and add a wineglass of white wine vinegar. Stir, then leave for 5 minutes – the milk will begin to curdle. Now pour it through a fine sieve or a colander lined with muslin. Allow the water to drain, then squeeze the remaining curd and chill in the fridge. Chop the cheese into thumb-sized pieces, fry in butter with a little chilli, garlic and sea salt and add to the curry.

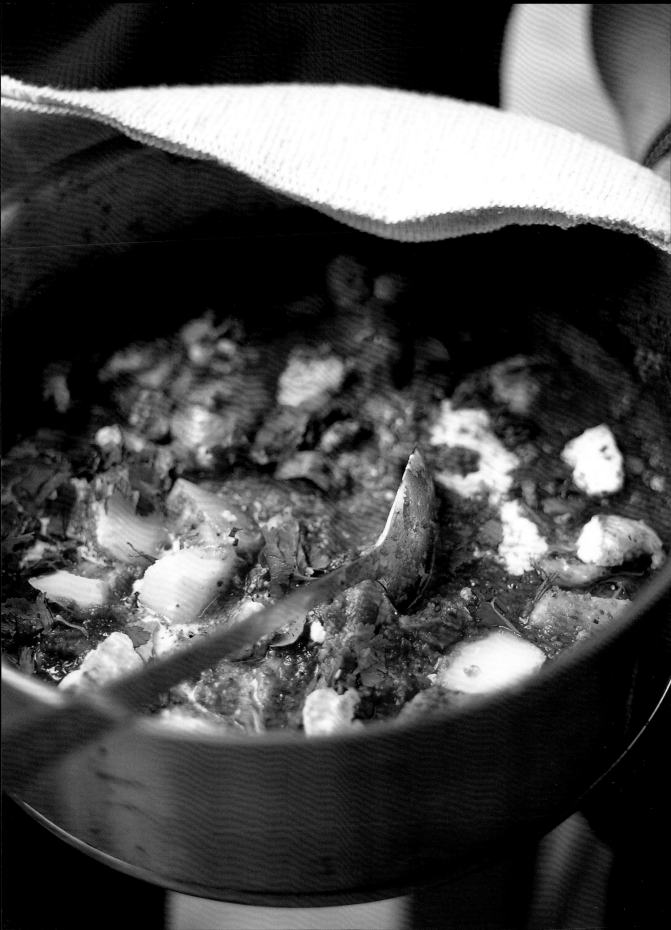

steaks, chops, fillets, legs & breasts, tenderloins, whole birds & half birds, cutlets, noisettes, medallions & all that malarkey

Absolutely everyone cooks these cuts of meat week in, week out. Pork, lamb, beef, chicken: we all cook them. And the idea of the marinades and rubs on pages 194–5 is to give you six possible ways to flavour them – to give you options other than the plain old grilled chop. When you have marinated or rubbed the chosen meat, grill, fry or roast it in a hot oven until perfectly cooked and leave to rest for 5 minutes.

marinades & rubs

Each of the following marinades and rubs will make enough to flavour 6 to 8 portions of meat (or fish!) – they're a fantastic way of adding flavour, taking it in a whole new direction. They're also great tenderizers, helping to break down any tough sinews.

The following flavours are just the tip of the iceberg. Feel free to vary them depending on what herbs, oils and ingredients you have available. I like to rub and massage the meat for a little while to really get the flavours in there. Sometimes I bash out pork chops so the surface area is a bit bigger, or even lightly score chicken to impart the flavour quicker. Marinate the meat for anything between 1 and 8 hours, but these marinades, when used on first-class pieces of meat, do work best when left all day. I wouldn't leave them for any longer than that. Get the meat in the marinade first thing before work and it will be ready to cook for dinner that night.

Rubs are great for simply and cheaply flavouring meat or fish as, generally, they're based around dried herbs and spices which are non-perishable. You can improvise and make up your own, but the three on page 195 are the ones I use all the time.

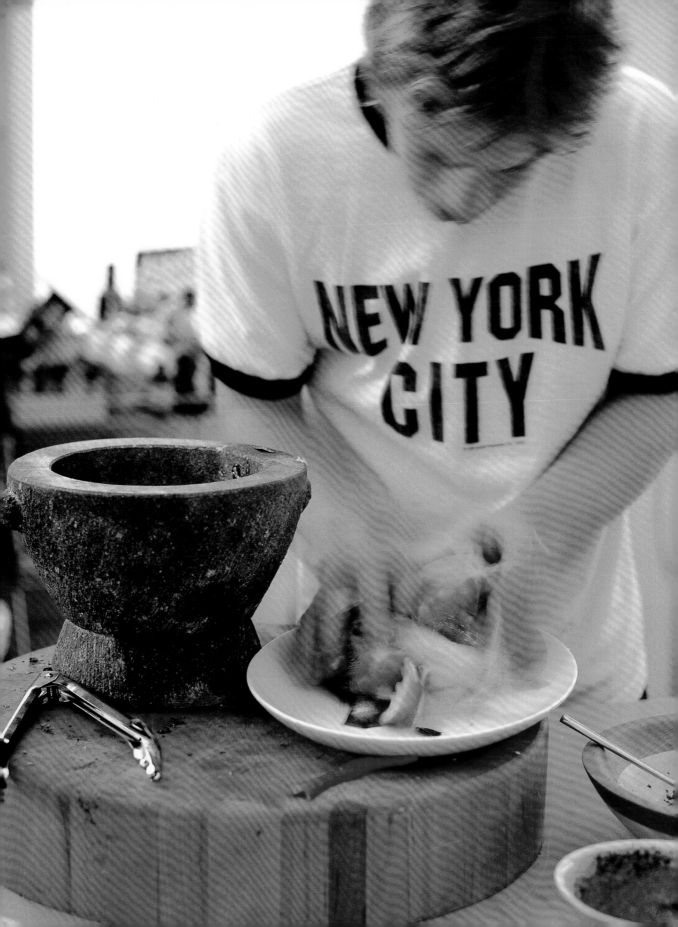

Asian marinade

2 sticks of lemongrass, crushed and bruised
1 small handful of kaffir lime leaves, torn
2 tablespoons low-salt soy sauce
2 cloves of garlic, crushed
5cm piece of fresh ginger, peeled and chopped
1 fresh red chilli, finely chopped
2 limes, halved, juiced and skin squashed
8 lugs of olive oil

Scrunch the ingredients together and rub over your
chosen meat or fish before leaving it to marinate.

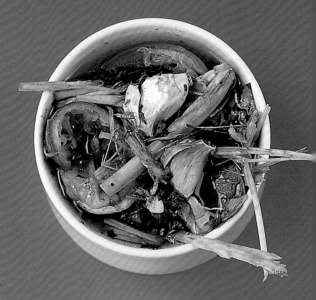

yoghurt, mint & lime marinade

1 × 500g tub of natural yoghurt
2 good handfuls of fresh mint, chopped
2 limes, zested and juiced
1 tablespoon coriander seeds, crushed
1 pinch of sea salt and black pepper
2 lugs of olive oil

Mix the ingredients together and rub over your chosen
meat before leaving it to marinate.

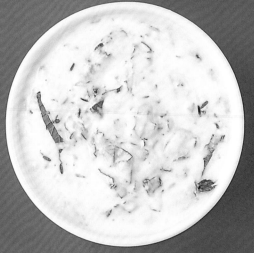

rosemary, garlic & lemon marinade

2 good handfuls of fresh rosemary, pounded
6 cloves of garlic, crushed
8 lugs of olive oil
3 lemons, juiced and skin squashed
1 pinch of black pepper

Mix the ingredients together and rub over your
chosen meat before leaving it to marinate.

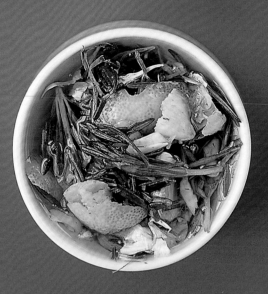

hot & fragrant rub

2 tablespoons fennel seeds
2 tablespoons cumin seeds
2 tablespoons coriander seeds
½ tablespoon fenugreek seeds
½ tablespoon black peppercorns
1 clove
½ a cinnamon stick
2 cardamom pods
1 pinch of sea salt and black pepper

Lightly toast all the ingredients in a pan over a gentle
heat before pounding or crushing into a fine powder.
Rub generously over your chosen meat.

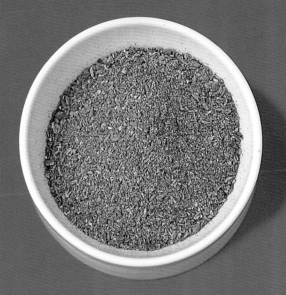

fennel seed, thyme & garlic rub

4 tablespoons fennel seeds
2 good handfuls of fresh thyme
2 cloves of garlic
1 fresh bay leaf, ripped
1 pinch of sea salt and black pepper

Pound all the ingredients together and rub generously
over your chosen meat.

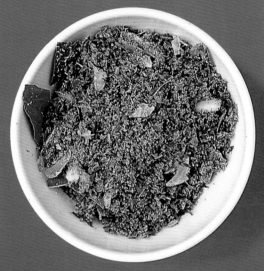

Cajun spicy rub

2 tablespoons paprika
2 tablespoons cayenne pepper
1 tablespoon black peppercorns, ground
2 cloves of garlic, peeled and crushed
3 tablespoons onion flakes
2 tablespoons dried oregano
1 pinch of sea salt

Pound all the ingredients together and rub
generously over your chosen meat.

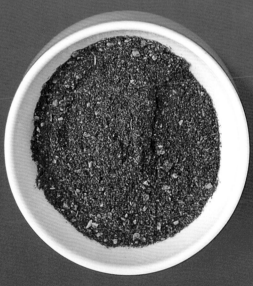

Botham burger

The good thing about burgers is you can make them thin and big, fat and big, or even turn them into meatballs. In the early days of the Cricketers, the pub where I grew up, I remember my dad used to serve a whopping great burger the size of a cricket ball topped with a huge amount of Cheddar cheese and homemade tomato relish. He very classily called it the Botham burger. That's what I love about Essex boys – sheer taste. Feel free to add extra spices if that's what takes your fancy, but here's a really solid basic beefburger recipe. I never thought when I became a chef that I would come back round to respecting the famous beefburger. Unfortunately it hasn't been on the pub's menu for years – what a shame. This might change Dad's mind.

serves 4
1kg minced beef
2 medium red onions, peeled and finely chopped
2 large eggs
1–2 handfuls of fresh breadcrumbs
1 tablespoon of coriander seeds, crushed
1 small pinch of cumin seeds, crushed
1 heaped teaspoon Dijon mustard

Preheat the oven to 230°C/450°F/gas 8. Mix and scrunch all the ingredients together with a pinch of sea salt and black pepper, using the breadcrumbs as required to bind and lighten the mixture. Divide into four, then gently and lightly mould and pack each burger together into a smallish cricket-ball-sized shape. Place in the oven and roast for 25 minutes, which should leave the middle slightly pink and the outsides nice and crispy. Serve with a griddled bun, a little salad, some gherkins, tomato salsa (see page 278), a pint of Guinness and a bottle of ketchup. Howzat!

CALORIES	FAT	SAT FAT	PROTEIN	CARBS	SUGAR	SALT	FIBRE
638kcal	43.7g	18g	54.1g	8.3g	4.7g	1.6g	2.1g

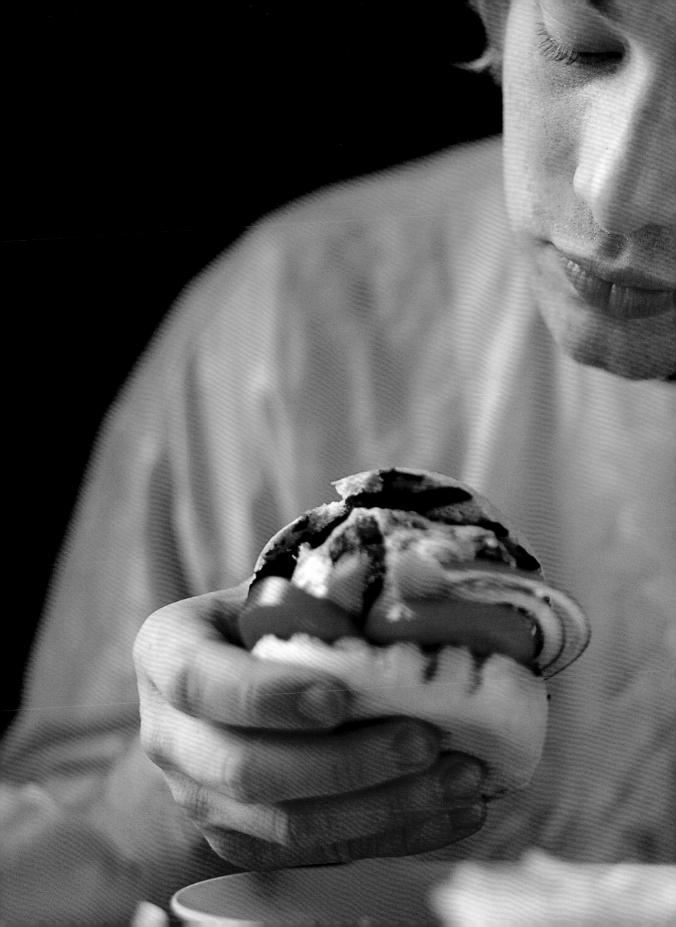

NARKA
NARKA
NA
N
N
NA

Geest

barry

vegetables

Nothing much has changed in the veg world over the last year and a half, since my first book, but I still believe a lot of good things are going to happen in general supermarkets and markets. I've heard a few rumours that certain supermarkets think they're going to be 90 per cent organic by 2005, which is great. I wouldn't worry about price either, because as we buy more British produce, grown properly as it used to be before we started cheating and churning it out, it will become nice and cheap so everyone can afford it. Also, the variety of vegetables like cabbages, potatoes and tomatoes, as well as salad leaves, is slowly getting better. Things that could only be bought for restaurant use before are now popping up in supermarkets and that's superb.

I have noticed people's curiosity about cooking becoming more intense, which is great. I think a lot of people are now beginning to learn a lot about cooking and are really enjoying it, though sometimes when I walk round the supermarket I see such a massive contrast in buyers and I'm sure that will always be the case. In general I'll see young couples with their trolleys full of quite interesting vegetables – asparagus, artichokes, rocket – talking and sometimes arguing about the best combinations and ways to cook their veg for dinner. I find it so interesting. Usually they have some really good ideas, but others are definite no-nos and I do feel the urge to go up to them and say, 'Excuse me, I'm Dr Naked Chef, can I possibly help?' But I know they would just turn round and say, 'Who are you? On yer bike, mate!' The main thing, though, is that they are interested and they are trying. However, I can never get over the mother with lots of pasty kids and a trolley full of Coke, crisps and tinned spaghetti hoops. I feel like kidnapping the kids and force-feeding them vegetables for a month to get some colour back into their cheeks. There's no such thing as a vegetable that is too flashy or complicated for a kid. In Italy it is so common to see two-year-olds nibbling on asparagus tips and dipping artichoke hearts in flavoured butters and sauces. They love it, it's good fun and it's bloomin' good for them. At the end of the day, their diet is only as good as that of their parents.

baked endive with thyme, orange juice, garlic & butter

Five years on from swearing that I'd never eat another Belgian endive again, I'm writing a recipe for one that I think is gorgeous. Hypocritical I know, but there you go.

serves 4
4 Belgian endive
3 generous knobs of unsalted butter
1 clove of garlic, peeled and finely chopped
1 good handful of fresh thyme, leaves picked
300ml fresh orange juice

Preheat the oven to 230°C/450°F/gas 8. Remove any discoloured outer leaves from the Belgian endive, if needed. Halve lengthways, then quarter each half. In a hot pan, fry the endive with the butter, garlic, thyme leaves and a pinch of sea salt and black pepper for about 4 minutes. Pour in the orange juice and allow to sizzle, then transfer it all to a dish, cover with tin foil and bake for 10 minutes. Now remove the tin foil and bake for a further 10 minutes. Taste and season before serving.

CALORIES	FAT	SAT FAT	PROTEIN	CARBS	SUGAR	SALT	FIBRE
152kcal	12.5g	8g	2.4g	7.6g	7.1g	0.5g	2.1g

baked fennel with garlic butter & vermouth

This dish is so quick. I made it the other day, chucked it together and it's really light and flavoursome. It goes fantastically well with any meat or fish.

serves 4
3 large heads of fennel
1 clove of garlic, peeled and finely sliced
3 large knobs of unsalted butter
2 wineglasses of vermouth (white wine also works)

Preheat the oven to 220°C/425°F/gas 7. Remove any discoloured parts of the fennel, then cut the tops off and slice finely, reserving the leaves. I normally slice each fennel from the top to the root, into about 4 pieces, but it's not that important. You can slice them finer and more delicately if you like. Throw all the ingredients except the reserved leaves into a baking dish and season with sea salt and black pepper. Rip off a piece of greaseproof paper, run it under cold water and scrunch it up to make it soft, then place it snugly over and around the fennel, not the actual dish. This bakes and steams the fennel at the same time – basically making it damn tasty! Bake for 20 minutes, or until tender. Sprinkle with the fennel leaves before serving.

CALORIES	FAT	SAT FAT	PROTEIN	CARBS	SUGAR	SALT	FIBRE
290kcal	12.9g	7.9g	3.5g	22g	2.8g	0.9g	8.1g

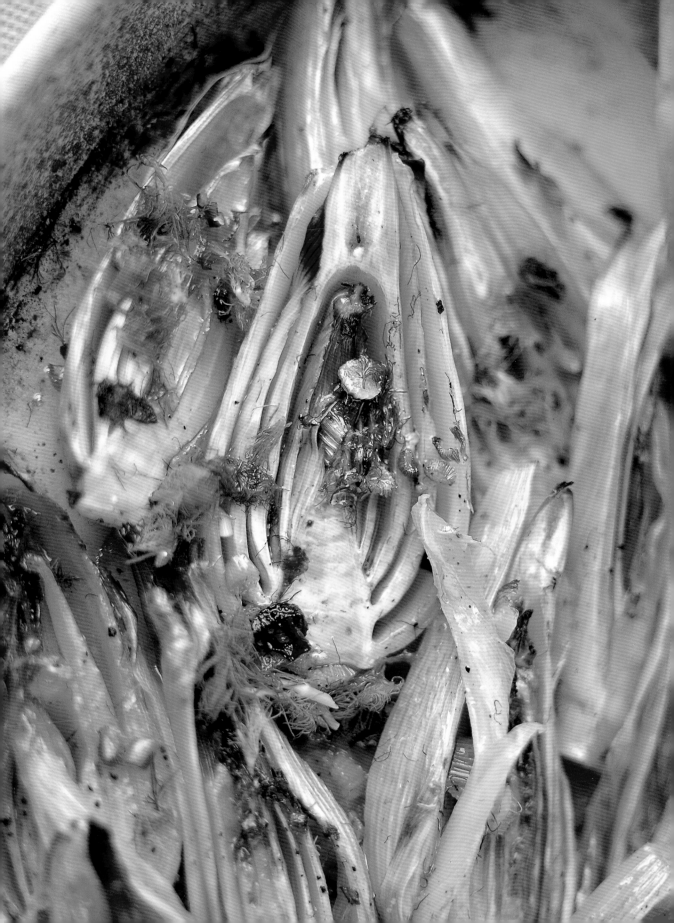

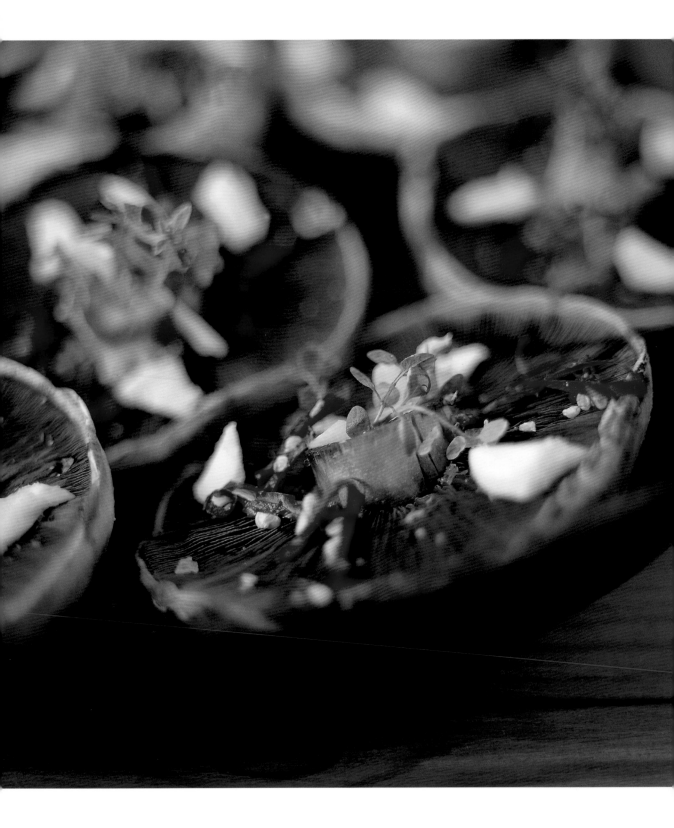

traybaked field mushrooms studded with garlic & rubbed with butter & thyme

In the restaurant we buy in some fantastic mushrooms, each with its own character, but they are very very expensive. With regard to mushrooms at home, stay a million miles away from the horrible boring button mushroom and go for the flat field mushroom. These vary in size, so I always buy ones as big as beer-mats. This recipe is absolutely fantastic, juicy and meaty.

serves 4

1 dried chilli
1 good handful of fresh thyme, leaves picked
2 cloves of garlic, peeled and finely sliced
1 lemon
6 good lugs of olive oil
4–8 flat field mushrooms, depending on size
1 knob of unsalted butter

Preheat the oven to 220°C/425°F/gas 7. Finely slice the dried chilli, then pound with the thyme leaves and a little garlic in a pestle and mortar. Squeeze in the lemon juice and add the oil. With your hand or a brush, rub the mushrooms all over with this mixture. Make sure all the flavoured oil is used up. Tightly pack the mushrooms together, bottom side up, in an ovenproof dish or roasting tray, and with a knife make 2 to 3 little slits randomly over each one. Insert a slice of the remaining garlic into each slit. Dot the butter over the mushrooms, season with sea salt and black pepper, and bake for around 15 to 25 minutes, depending on the size of your mushrooms – taste one and see – they should be soft, slightly coloured and damn juicy. Great served with steak and chips, ripped into a warm salad, chopped into ravioli, sliced and tossed with pasta and a bit of cream . . . nice one.

vegetables

CALORIES	FAT	SAT FAT	PROTEIN	CARBS	SUGAR	SALT	FIBRE
318kcal	34.4g	6.9g	1.6g	0.9g	0.2g	0.7g	0.5g

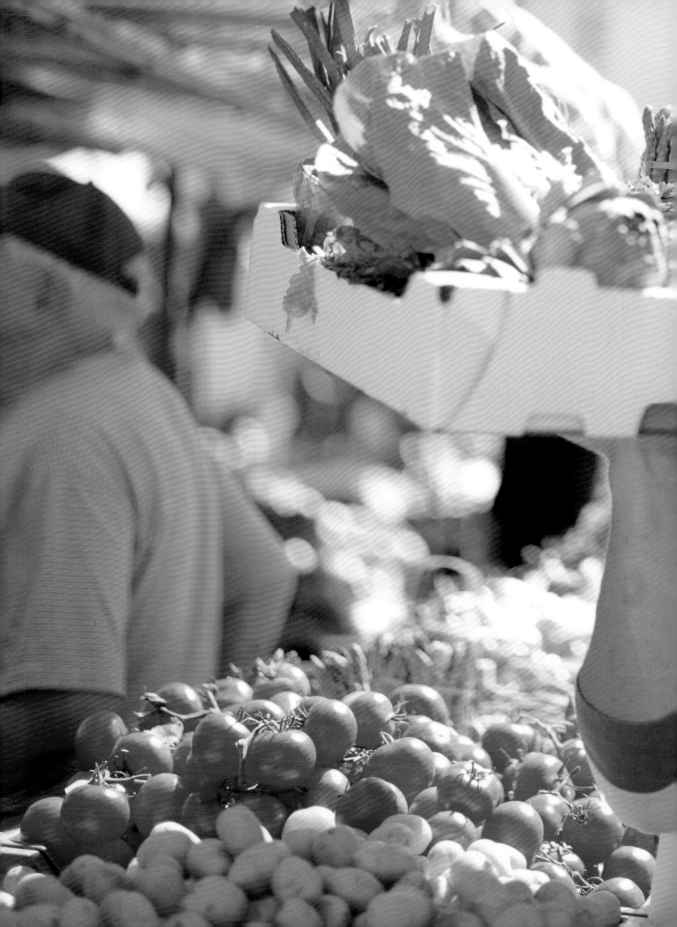

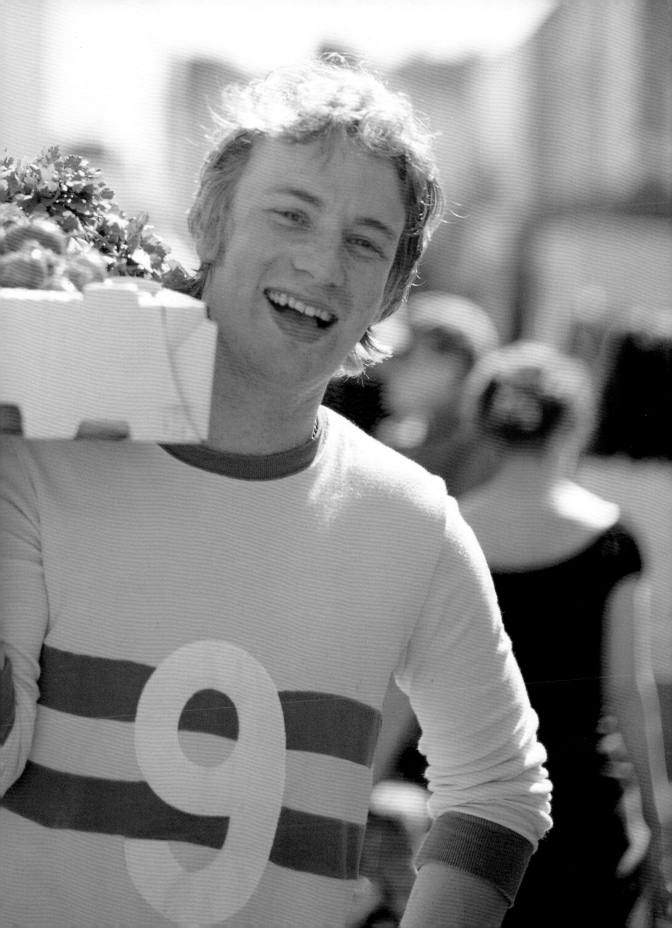

baked Jerusalem artichokes, breadcrumbs, thyme & lemon

This dish is absolutely spanking in the middle of your table for a Sunday roast or with a grilled bit of chicken or a pork chop. The breadcrumbs and thyme become crispy on top, giving the dish a really sexy texture of soft artichoke and crisp topping.

serves 6
250ml double cream or crème fraîche
1 lemon
2 cloves of garlic, peeled and finely chopped
1 good handful of fresh thyme, leaves picked and chopped
3 handfuls of freshly grated Parmesan cheese
1kg Jerusalem artichokes, peeled and sliced
  as thick as a pencil
2 good handfuls of fresh breadcrumbs
olive oil

Preheat the oven to 220°C/425°F/gas 7. Mix the cream, lemon juice, garlic, half the thyme leaves and most of the Parmesan together, and season well with sea salt and black pepper. Throw in the sliced Jerusalem artichokes. Mix well and place everything in a baking dish.

Mix the breadcrumbs with the rest of the thyme and Parmesan and some salt and pepper. Sprinkle the flavoured breadcrumbs over the artichokes and drizzle with a little oil. Bake for 45 minutes, or until the artichokes are tender and the breadcrumbs are beautifully golden and crisp.

vegetables

CALORIES	FAT	SAT FAT	PROTEIN	CARBS	SUGAR	SALT	FIBRE
367kcal	28.4g	16.9g	9.5g	22.4g	3.8g	0.7g	6.2g

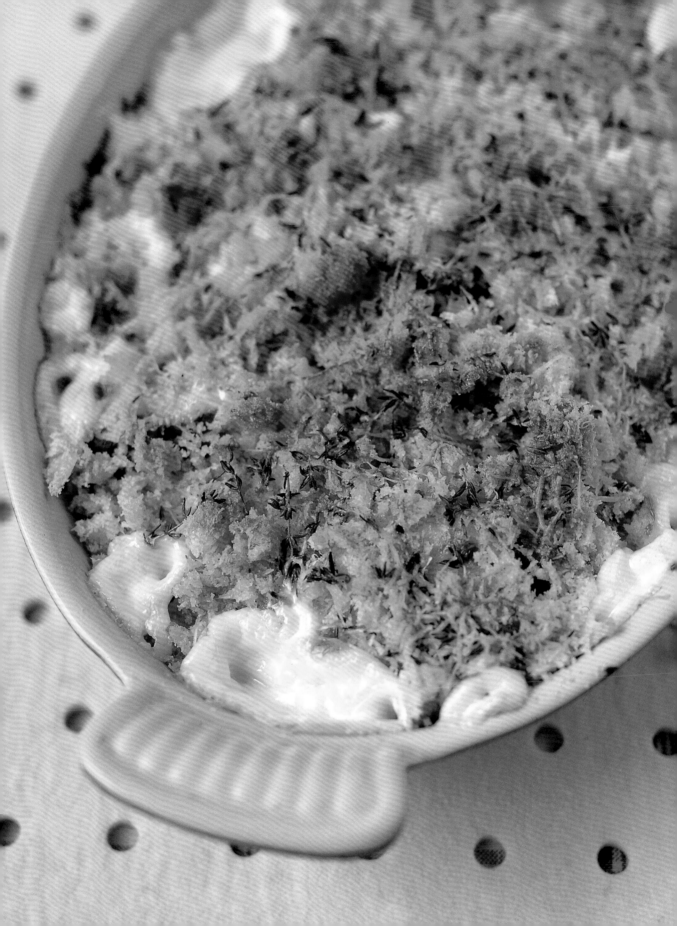

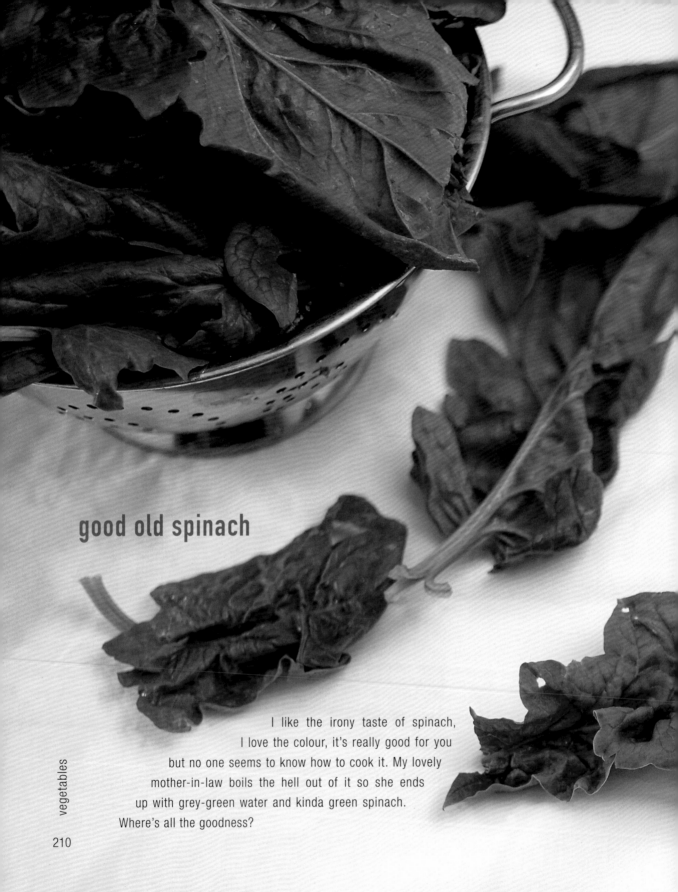

good old spinach

I like the irony taste of spinach,
I love the colour, it's really good for you
but no one seems to know how to cook it. My lovely
mother-in-law boils the hell out of it so she ends
up with grey-green water and kinda green spinach.
Where's all the goodness?

In the water. So forget everything you know about cooking spinach, this is the way we do it from now on. Either pick or buy spinach on the stalk, which you should wash well, sometimes two or three times but that's not the end of the world. If you've got lovely young leaves, leave them on the stalk and just pick the outer leaves off. Or, as most of us do, buy packs of prewashed baby spinach from the supermarket – how convenient. Here are four brilliant ways with spinach. You can also use Swiss chard or Savoy cabbage in place of spinach.

the simplest spinach with nutmeg & butter

serves 4

Drizzle a little olive oil into a hot pan or wok, sway the pan about and add 4 huge handfuls of spinach. This will look like a lot, but it will soon cook down. It will sizzle a bit, so just stand by it and turn it over every 5 seconds. After about 30 seconds it will begin to wilt and hopefully only a little water will start to cook out of the spinach (if there is a lot then pour a little away). Add 3 big knobs of unsalted butter and grate in about 12 scrapings of nutmeg, to taste. Mix, season with sea salt and black pepper, and serve – the butter and water should mix together giving you just enough natural sauce to bind everything together.

CALORIES	FAT	SAT FAT	PROTEIN	CARBS	SUGAR	SALT	FIBRE
128kcal	13.6g	8g	1.3g	0.2g	0.1g	0.6g	0.5g

spinach & porcini mushrooms with rosemary & lemon

serves 4

Dried porcini mushrooms are everywhere now – their flavour is extreme and extraordinary. A small pack (30g) is more than enough for this recipe. Just cover the porcini mushrooms with boiling water and soak for 15 minutes. Keeping the liquor to one side, fry the mushrooms with 2 knobs of unsalted butter, 1 chopped clove of garlic and around 1 tablespoon of finely chopped fresh rosemary. Fry for 4 minutes, then gently pour in around half the soaking liquor – I say gently because sometimes a little grit falls to the bottom, which you don't want. Simmer the mushrooms until the butter and liquor have reduced just enough to coat them, then plonk in 4 huge handfuls of spinach and mix round until the spinach is vibrant green and wilted. Season to taste with a squeeze of lemon juice, sea salt and black pepper. An excellent filling for vegetarian cannelloni with a little ricotta.

CALORIES	FAT	SAT FAT	PROTEIN	CARBS	SUGAR	SALT	FIBRE
109kcal	8.8g	5.3g	3.7g	3.7g	1.2g	0.2g	1.4g

spring onions, sweet peas, white wine & spinach

serves 4

In a pot slowly fry a handful of finely chopped spring onions for a couple of minutes in a lug of olive oil and a knob of unsalted butter, then add 2 handfuls of fresh or frozen peas and cook for another couple of minutes before adding a good glass of white wine. Bring to the boil and simmer for a few minutes before adding 4 huge handfuls of spinach. Turn this over and cook until the spinach is wilted. Add 2 knobs of unsalted butter and season well to taste.

CALORIES	FAT	SAT FAT	PROTEIN	CARBS	SUGAR	SALT	FIBRE
192kcal	15.4g	8.3g	2.6g	3g	1.6g	0.2g	0.8g

steamed spinach with coconut rice

serves 4

1 × 400ml tin of light coconut milk

300g long-grain rice

4 tablespoons low-salt soy sauce

2 tablespoons extra virgin olive oil

4 handfuls of baby spinach

Place the coconut milk in a pan and top up with enough water to cook the rice in. Bring to the boil, add a pinch of sea salt and the rice. Cook until the rice is tender, then drain in a colander. Pour a little more water into the pan and put it back on the heat. Place the colander over the pan and simmer the water to steam the rice, making it light and fluffy. Place in a warm serving bowl, add the soy sauce and extra virgin olive oil and stir in the spinach. The heat from the rice will cook the spinach in a matter of minutes, keeping it lovely and green and retaining all its goodness.

CALORIES	FAT	SAT FAT	PROTEIN	CARBS	SUGAR	SALT	FIBRE
409kcal	13.4g	6.4g	7.8g	68.1g	3g	1.7g	1.6g

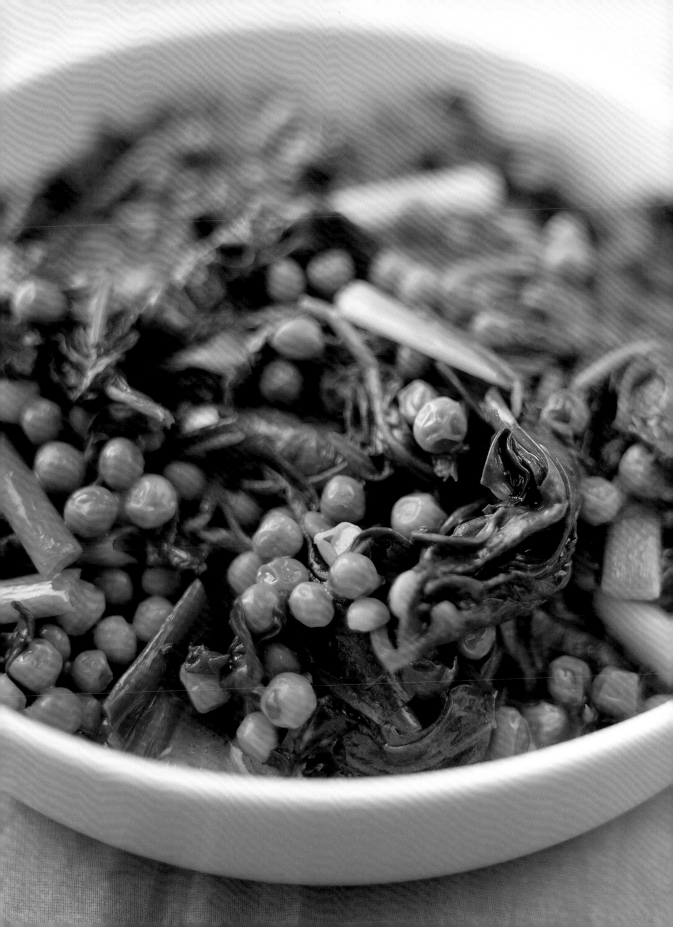

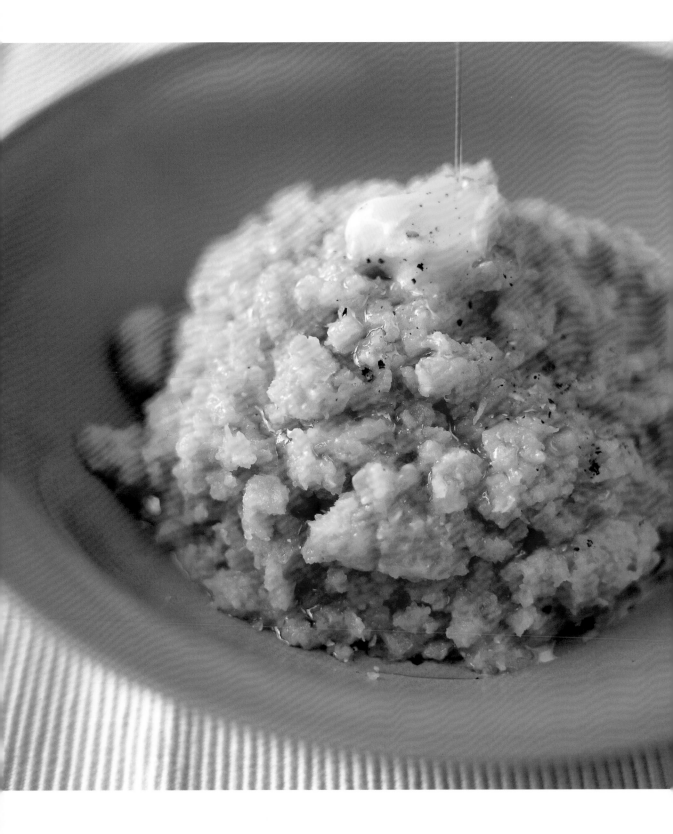

good old mashed veg

This is a gutsy veg dish which just about everyone loves. My missus makes me fantastic mashed vegetables, beautifully seasoned and drizzled with olive oil – the only thing is, they are meant to be separate servings of boiled carrots and new potatoes! So if you, too, are prone to overcooking your veg, just mash it all together.

serves 4
2kg root vegetables, such as celeriac, potatoes,
   swede, parsnips, carrots, Jerusalem artichokes
extra virgin olive oil or unsalted butter

Feel free to use any single vegetable or a mixture of your favourites. Simply peel them, chop them into golf-ball sized pieces, place in boiling salted water and cook until nice and tender. Drain in a colander before placing the veg back in the pan and mashing with a potato masher. Make it as smooth or as chunky as you like. Season carefully with sea salt and black pepper, then enrich the flavour with extra virgin olive oil or unsalted butter, or both, to taste.

Once cooked, the mash can be kept warm in a bowl covered with tin foil over simmering water. This is handy when cooking for a dinner party, as you can get one lot of veg done and nicely out of the way.

vegetables

CALORIES	FAT	SAT FAT	PROTEIN	CARBS	SUGAR	SALT	FIBRE
222kcal	2.3g	0.4g	6.1g	47.1g	20.5g	0.6g	16.3g

baked beetroot with balsamic vinegar, marjoram & garlic

Beetroot is a fantastic veg, which is great served with white fish such as grilled monkfish, or with beef carpaccio (see page 175), or as part of an antipasti plate along with some tasty beans, sliced prosciutto and tomato-rubbed crostini. If you're lucky enough to buy beetroots with their leaves, remove them, keep them and use like baby spinach – they taste amazing.

serves 4
450g fresh raw beetroots, preferably golf-ball size, scrubbed
10 cloves of garlic, unpeeled and squashed
1 handful of fresh marjoram or sweet oregano, leaves picked
10 tablespoons balsamic vinegar
6 tablespoons olive oil

Preheat the oven to 200°C/400°F/gas 6. Tear off around 1.5 metres of tin foil and fold it in half to give you double thickness. If you can only get larger beetroots halve them to speed up their cooking time, otherwise use them whole. Place them in the middle of the tin foil with the garlic and marjoram leaves, season generously with sea salt and black pepper, then fold the sides in to the middle. Before you seal the tin foil, add the vinegar and oil. Scrunch or fold the tin foil together to seal at the top. Roast for around 1 hour, or until tender. Serve in the bag at the table – lovely.

CALORIES	FAT	SAT FAT	PROTEIN	CARBS	SUGAR	SALT	FIBRE
282kcal	19.7g	2.8g	3.4g	22.9g	20.1g	0.7g	2.4g

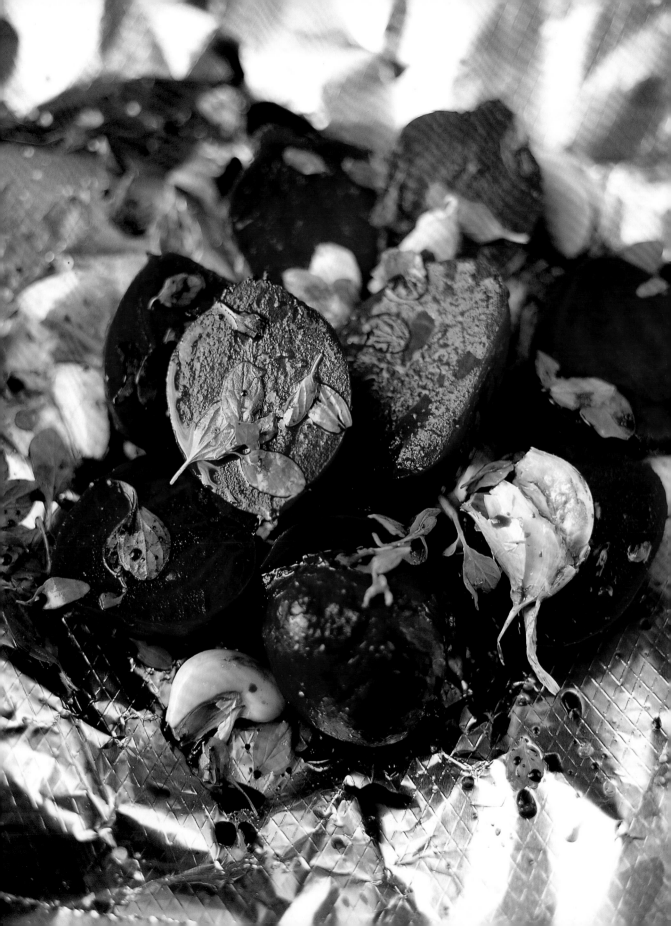

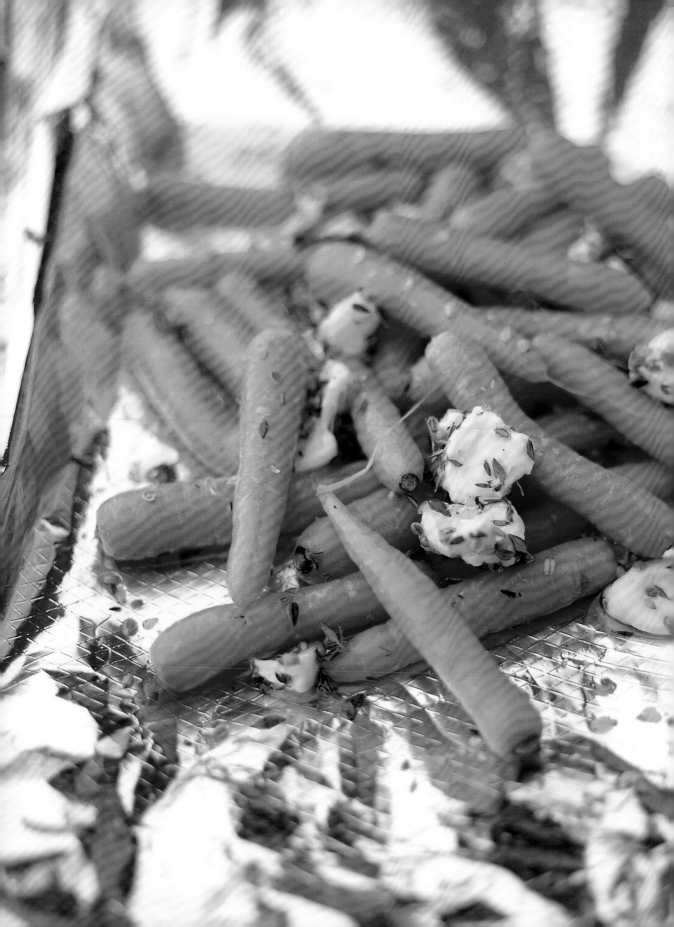

baked carrots with cumin, thyme, butter & Chardonnay

I love this dish made with baby carrots, but feel free to use fat old ones sliced at an angle if you please. Butter and wine make a fantastic sauce which just makes it for me. Serve with anything you like.

serves 4
450g baby carrots, scrubbed
½ teaspoon cumin seeds, crushed
1 handful of fresh thyme, leaves picked
4 knobs of unsalted butter
1 glass of Chardonnay

Preheat the oven to 220°C/425°F/gas 7. Tear off around 1.5 metres of tin foil and fold it in half to give you double thickness. Place everything but the wine in the middle of the tin foil. Bring up the sides and pour in the white wine. Season well with sea salt and black pepper, then fold or scrunch the tin foil together to seal. Roast for 45 minutes, or until the carrots are tender. Cook for longer if the carrots are bigger than baby ones.

vegetables

CALORIES	FAT	SAT FAT	PROTEIN	CARBS	SUGAR	SALT	FIBRE
222kcal	17.1g	10.5g	0.9g	9.5g	8.5g	0.6g	4.7g

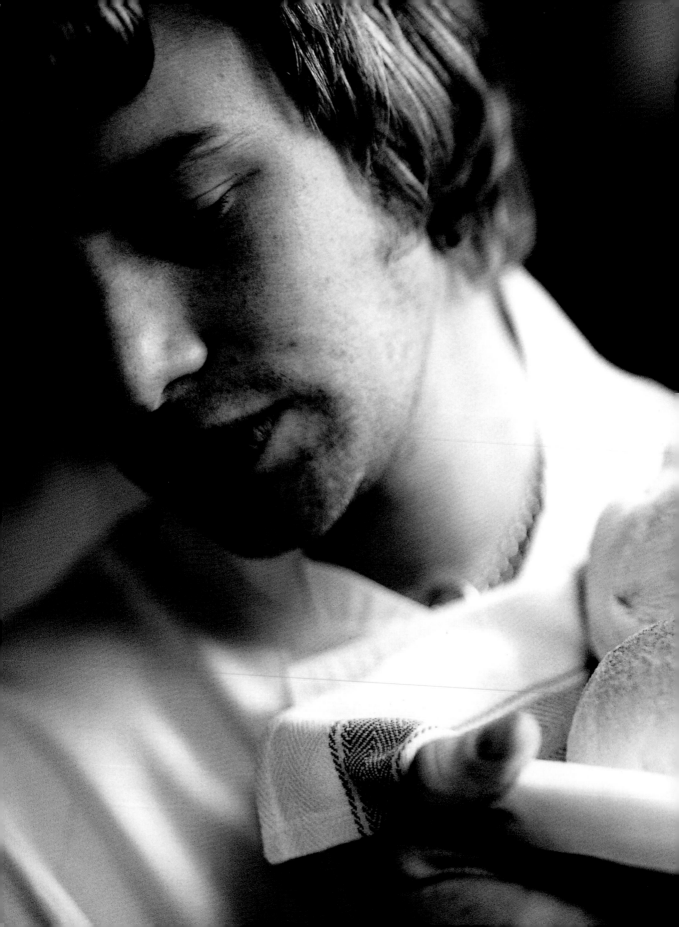

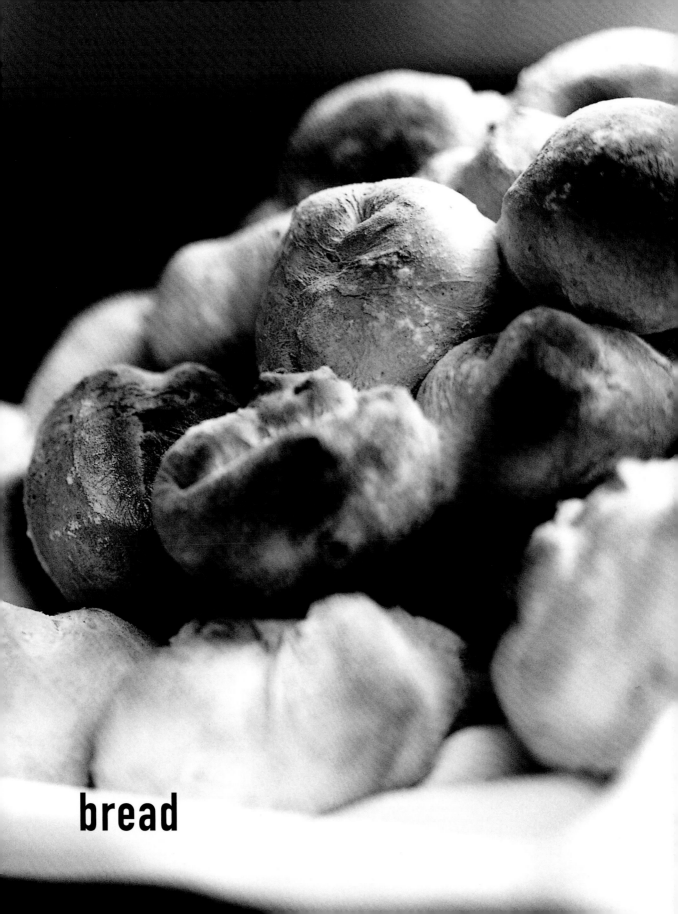

bread

basic bread recipe

30g fresh yeast or 3 × 7g sachets dried yeast
30g runny honey (or sugar)
1kg strong bread flour, plus extra for dusting

Stage 1

Dissolve the yeast and honey (or sugar) in 300ml of tepid water.

Stage 2

On a clean surface or in a large bowl, make a pile of the flour and 10g of sea salt.
Make a well in the centre and pour in all the dissolved yeast mixture. With 4 fingers of
one hand, make circular movements from the centre moving outwards, slowly bringing
in more and more of the flour until all the yeast mixture is soaked up. Pour another
300ml of the tepid water into the centre and gradually incorporate all the flour to make
a moist dough. (Certain flours may need a little more water, so don't be afraid to adjust
the quantities if needed.)

Stage 3

Kneading! This is the best bit, just rolling, pushing and folding the dough over and over
for 5 minutes. This develops the gluten and the structure of the dough. If any of the
dough sticks to your hands, just rub them together with a little extra flour.

Stage 4

Flour both your hands well, and lightly flour the top of the dough. Make it into a
roundish shape and place on a baking tray. Deeply score the dough with a knife —
allowing it to relax and prove with ease. Leave it to prove until it's doubled in size.
Ideally you want a warm, draught-free place for the quickest prove, for example near a
warm cooker, in the airing cupboard or just in a warmish room, and you can even cover
it with a clean damp tea towel if you want to speed things up. This proving process
improves the flavour and texture of the dough and should take around 40 minutes to
1 hour 30 minutes, depending on the conditions.

bread

CALORIES	FAT	SAT FAT	PROTEIN	CARBS	SUGAR	SALT	FIBRE
155kcal	0.6g	0.1g	5.1g	34.7g	1.1g	0.2g	1.4g

THESE VALUES ARE BASED ON A 50G SLICE

Stage 5

When the dough has doubled in size you need to knock the air out of it by bashing it around for a minute. Now you can shape it into whatever shape is required – round, flat, filled, trayed up, tinned up or whatever – and leave it to prove for a second time until it doubles in size again. The important thing is not to lose your confidence now. Don't feel a need to rush through this, because the second proving time will give you the lovely, delicate soft texture that we all love in fresh bread.

Stage 6

Now it's time to cook your loaf. After all your hard work, don't spoil your efforts. You want to keep all the air inside the loaf, so don't knock it. Gently place it in the preheated oven, don't slam the door. Bake according to the time and temperature given in the recipe variations which follow. You can tell if your bread is cooked by tapping its bottom (if it's in a tin you'll have to take it out). If it sounds hollow it's cooked, if it doesn't then pop it back in for a little longer. Place it on a rack to cool. You're going to love this bread!

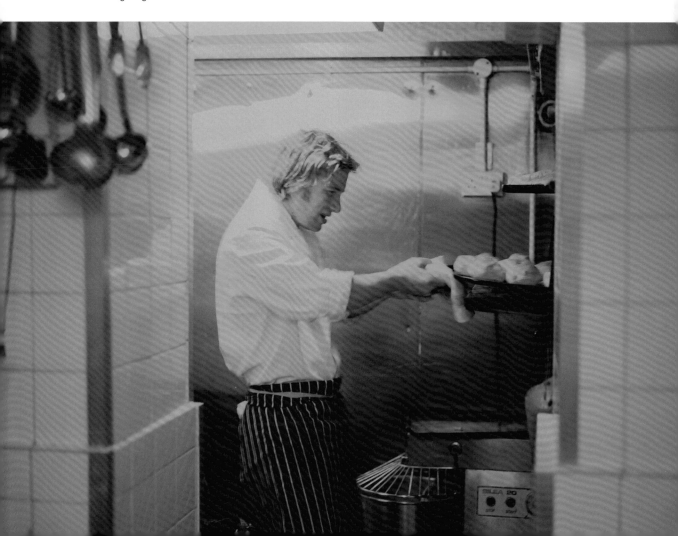

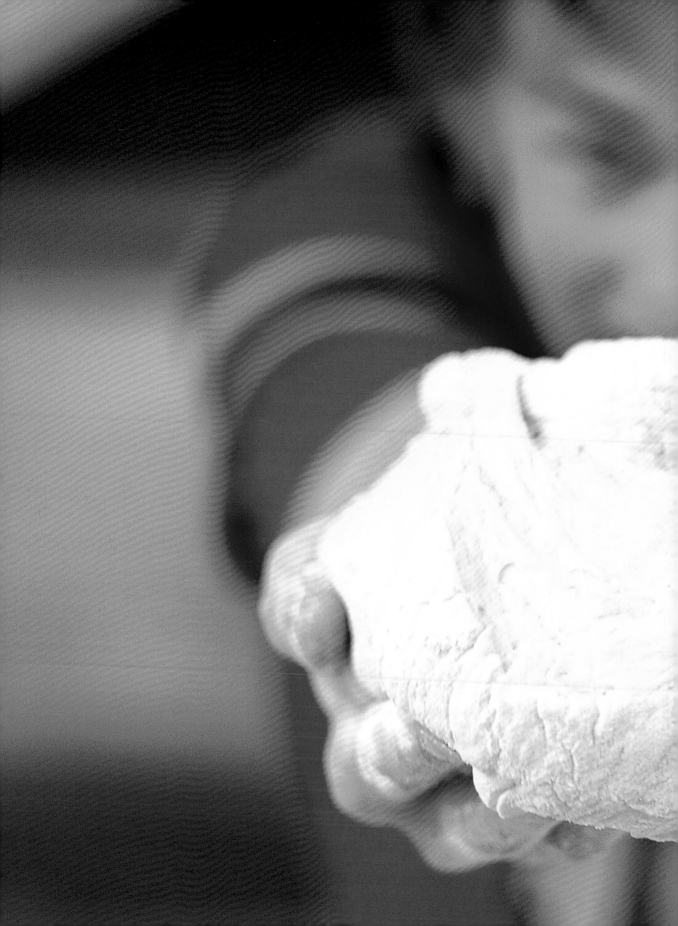

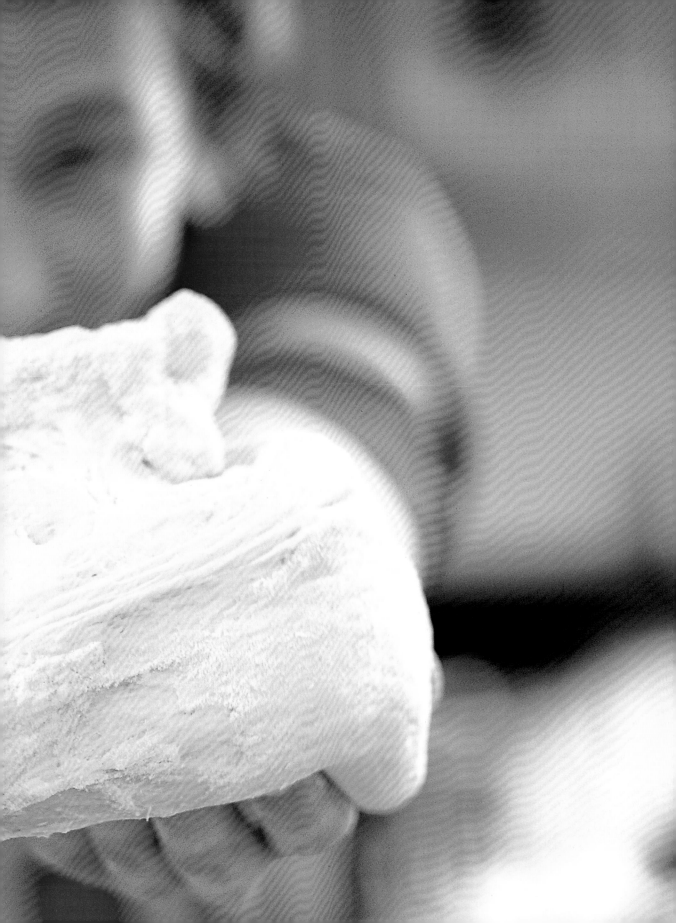

chocolate twister bread

1 × basic bread recipe (see pages 222–3)
200g unsalted butter (at room temperature)
200g hazelnuts, lightly roasted and crushed or broken up
300g of quality dark chocolate (70%), smashed up or grated

At Stage 5 of the basic bread recipe, divide the dough into 2 equal parts. After proving for the second time, take each piece of dough and push out into a squarish shape on a floured board. Then roll out to about 18cm wide. At this point, roll the other way and keep rolling to achieve a long rectangle about ½cm thick – it doesn't have to be exact. Using a knife, spread the butter thinly across the dough. Sprinkle over the hazelnuts and chocolate and roll up across the width like a Swiss roll. Cut across into 2cm wide slices. Place the slices next to each other on a greased baking tray, cut side upwards (rather like Chelsea buns), with small gaps in between. Bake in a preheated oven at 200°C/400°F/gas 6 for around 20 minutes. Allow to cool for 20 minutes before eating with a glass of cold milk.

bread

CALORIES	FAT	SAT FAT	PROTEIN	CARBS	SUGAR	SALT	FIBRE
509kcal	26.9g	12g	11g	58.1g	7.8g	0.3g	5.1g

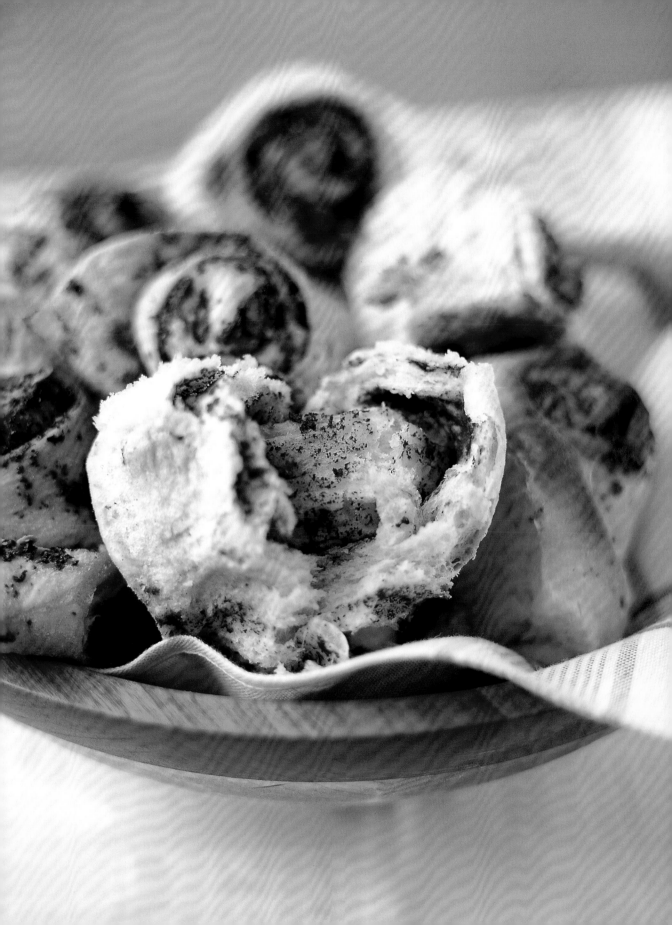

fruit loaf

Don't worry if you haven't got a tin to make this in. Simply shape into a round, place on a flour-dusted tray and score in a criss-cross fashion.

1 × basic bread recipe (see pages 222–3)
1 pinch of ground cinnamon
1 clove, ground
200g dried apricots
100g dried dates
200g dried raisins

Place the spices and fruit in a food processor or chop very finely. Scrunch into the dough mixture at Stage 2 of the basic bread recipe, possibly holding back a little water from the recipe, as residual water in dried fruit varies. Once you have a good dough consistency, carry on as normal until Stage 5.

After knocking all the air out of the dough, pack it into an appropriately sized greased and floured bread tin. The unproved dough should just underfill the tin, so at the end of Stage 5, when it's proved for the second time, the bread will have doubled in size and will be a whopping great light and fruity blooming bloomer. Lovely. Bake in a preheated oven for around 50 minutes at 200°C/400°F/gas 6, then remove from the tin and put the loaf back in the oven for a final 10 minutes, or until it sounds hollow when tapped. Allow to cool for 30 minutes.

CALORIES	FAT	SAT FAT	PROTEIN	CARBS	SUGAR	SALT	FIBRE
222kcal	0.6g	0.2g	6.4g	50.8g	14.8g	0.2g	2.2g

THESE VALUES ARE BASED ON A 50G SLICE

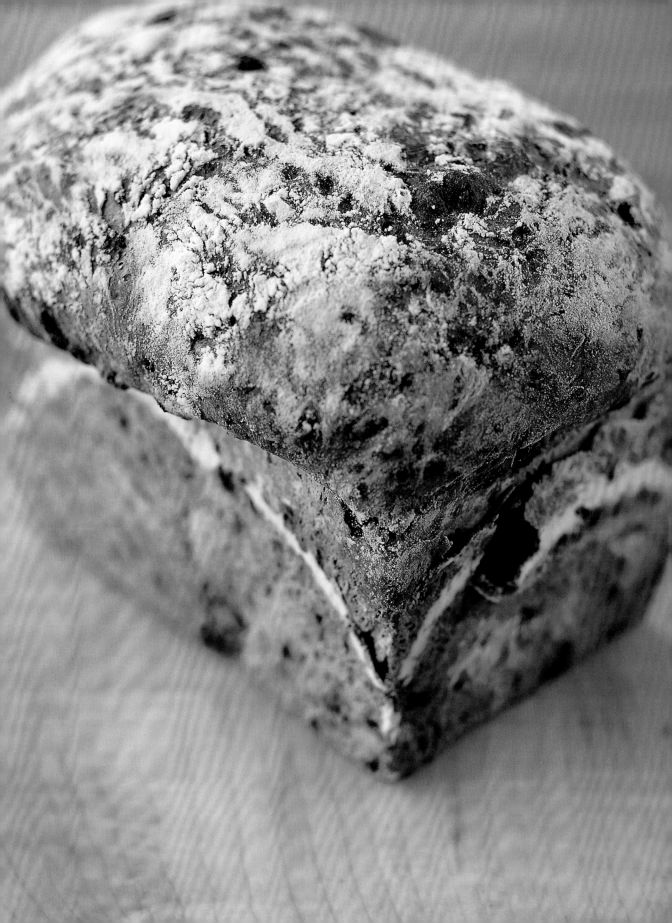

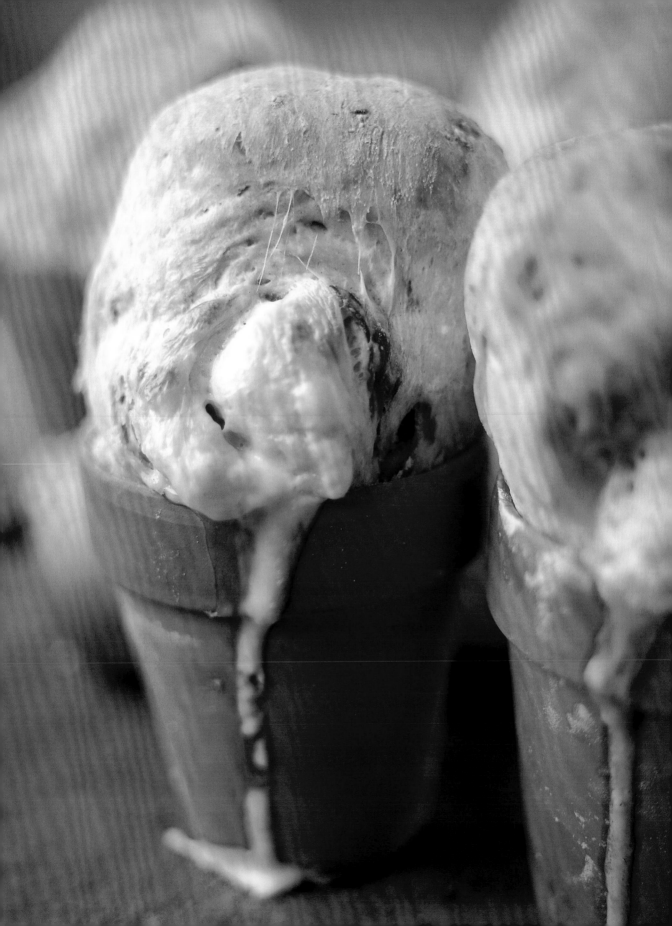

Gennaro bread

This is a bread very similar to one my mate Gennaro Contaldo used to make with the leftover, slightly dried-up, unwanted cheese and remaining prosciutto. The bread looks fantastic baked in unglazed, clean little terracotta pots but, quite frankly, you can cook this bread as rolls or as a loaf. Adjust the cooking time accordingly.

1 × basic bread recipe (see pages 222–3)
400g mixed cheese, such as Parmesan, fontina, Taleggio and
  a little Gorgonzola, grated or broken up
4 large egg yolks
10 slices of prosciutto, torn up
1 handful of fresh basil, torn

At Stage 2 of the basic bread recipe, mix in all the ingredients and carry on through to Stage 5, when you should divide the dough into 8 balls. I like to put them into 8 small, greased and floured, terracotta plant pots. Flour the top and prove until doubled in size. Bake in a preheated oven for around 30 minutes at 220°C/425°F/gas 7.

bread

231

CALORIES	FAT	SAT FAT	PROTEIN	CARBS	SUGAR	SALT	FIBRE
709kcal	21.4g	11.1g	33g	102.6g	3.9g	2.4g	4.1g

pizzas

Pizza bases are great to make, as they only need to prove once. The recipe below makes enough for 4 pizza bases (serves 8). Top with one of my three suggested toppings or some of your own favourite ones.

pizza base
1 × basic bread recipe (see pages 222–3)

At Stage 5 of the basic bread recipe, divide the dough into 4 pieces and simply roll each into a large, plate-sized, slightly irregular round shape about ½cm thick, using a rolling pin. Once you've added your chosen topping, place the pizza directly on to the bars of a preheated oven and bake for around 5 to 7 minutes at full whack (240°C/475°F/gas 9), or until the topping has melted and the pizza base is golden.

olive, tomato, rocket, Parmesan & mozzarella pizza

Halve and deseed 8 ripe plum tomatoes and dice them. Place in a bowl with 2 good handfuls of destoned olives. Season with sea salt and black pepper, a touch of olive oil and a splash of red wine vinegar. Spread this on to each pizza base, then sprinkle with pieces of mozzarella. Bake as above, then remove from the oven and sprinkle with some lightly dressed rocket and a good shaving of Parmesan cheese.

mushroom, mozzarella, thyme & spicy sausage meat pizza

Slice up 6 fat field mushrooms and fry with a good handful of fresh thyme leaves and some chopped garlic in a little olive oil until golden. Season well with sea salt and black pepper and remove from the heat. Add a little olive oil and spread the mushrooms evenly over each pizza base. Split the skins of 4 spicy sausages and sprinkle very small pieces of the meat on top of the mushrooms. Scatter with a little chopped fresh chilli, add a little mozzarella or other melting cheese – Taleggio or fontina – and bake in the oven as above.

mozzarella, prosciutto & basil pizza

Rub the pizza bases with olive oil and randomly scatter with pieces of buffalo mozzarella. Rip over some fresh basil and a couple of nice slices of prosciutto or Parma ham. Bake in the oven as above and serve with grated fresh Parmesan.

CALORIES	FAT	SAT FAT	PROTEIN	CARBS	SUGAR	SALT	FIBRE
555kcal	9.1g	4.8g	21.3g	103.6g	5.2g	1.3g	4.7g

THESE VALUES ARE BASED ON THE OLIVE, TOMATO, ROCKET, PARMESAN & MOZZARELLA PIZZA

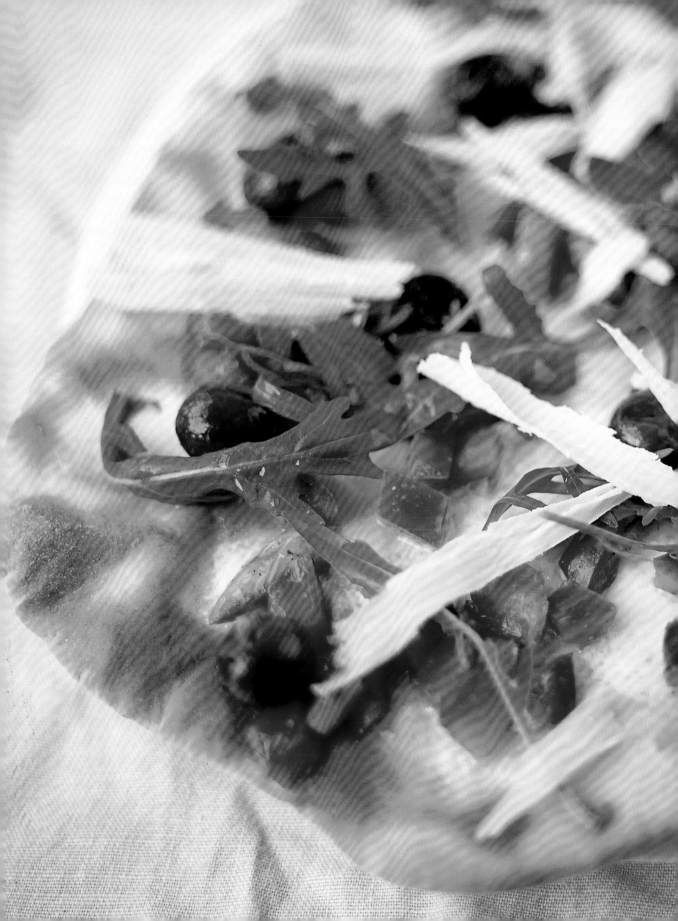

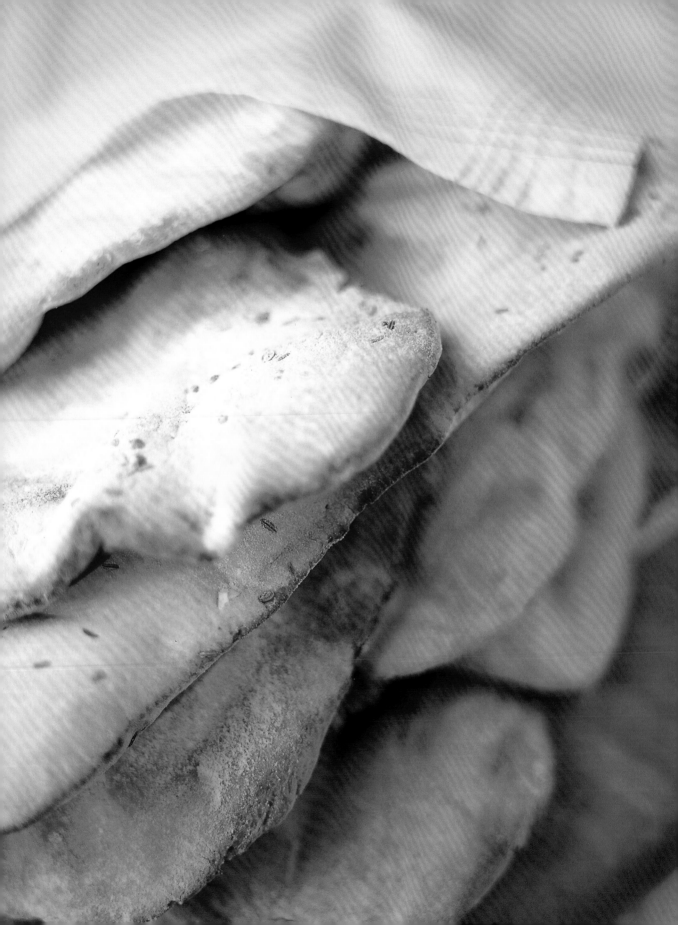

chickpea Moroccan flatbread

A very quick bread to make as it only needs one prove. Great for filling with salad, salsas and grilled meats, and especially tasty cooked on barbecues. Also great served with all the tapas recipes (see pages 36–51).

1 × basic bread recipe (see pages 222–3)
1 tablespoon of cumin seeds, lightly cracked
1 tablespoon of coriander seeds, lightly cracked
1 × 400g tin of chickpeas, drained and mashed

At Stage 2 of the basic bread recipe, mix in the cumin seeds, coriander seeds and chickpeas and carry on through the recipe as normal until Stage 5, when you should divide the batch of dough into 10 pieces. Roll out each of these to ½cm thick and gently pull out into a slightly irregular oval shape. Cook 1 or 2 at a time, depending on how big your oven is, straight away without a second prove, directly on the bars of a preheated oven at 230°C/450°F/gas 8. They take about 4 minutes to cook and puff up beyond belief. Allow to cool slightly for a couple of minutes before eating.

CALORIES	FAT	SAT FAT	PROTEIN	CARBS	SUGAR	SALT	FIBRE
391kcal	2g	0.4g	13.8g	85.3g	2.9g	0.4g	4.7g

slashed cheese, chilli & paprika flatbread

Great with salads and salamis. Oh, and roast chicken.

1 × basic bread recipe (see pages 222–3)
150g goat's cheese, broken up
150g freshly grated Parmesan cheese
1 heaped tablespoon paprika
4–6 dried red chillies, crumbled

Add all the ingredients at Stage 2 of the basic bread recipe, then carry on through to Stage 5, when, after knocking out the air, you should divide the bread into 2 pieces and roll them out in an irregular elongated triangle shape, about ½cm thick. Slash the bread about 5 or 6 times and stretch it open to expose the gaps. Place on a large baking tray and allow to prove for around 20 minutes before baking in a preheated oven at 220°C/425°F/gas 7 for 15 to 20 minutes, or until golden. Allow to cool for 10 minutes before eating.

CALORIES	FAT	SAT FAT	PROTEIN	CARBS	SUGAR	SALT	FIBRE
281kcal	5.8g	3.5g	12.4g	48.4g	1.9g	0.6g	2.2g

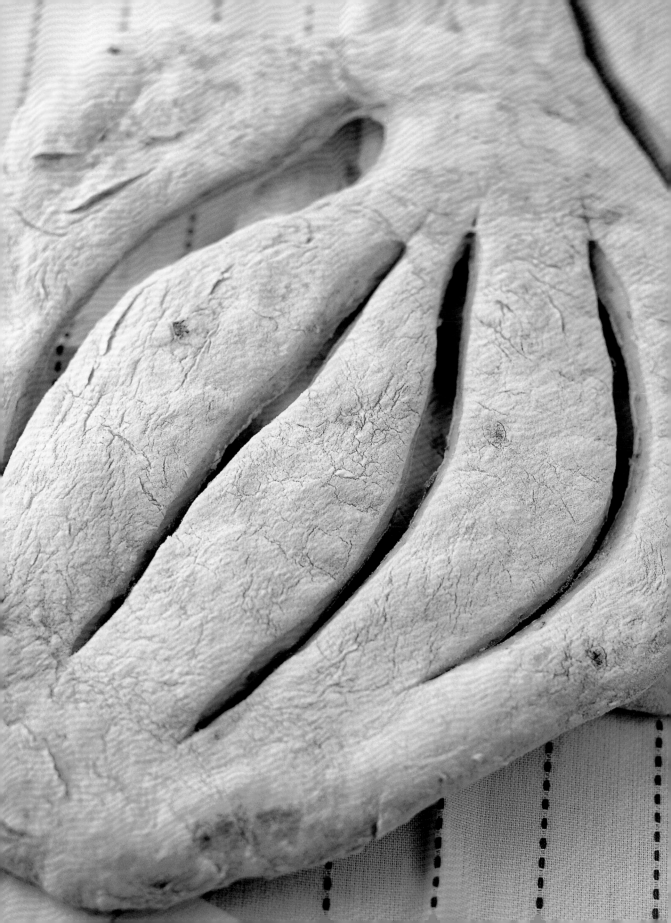

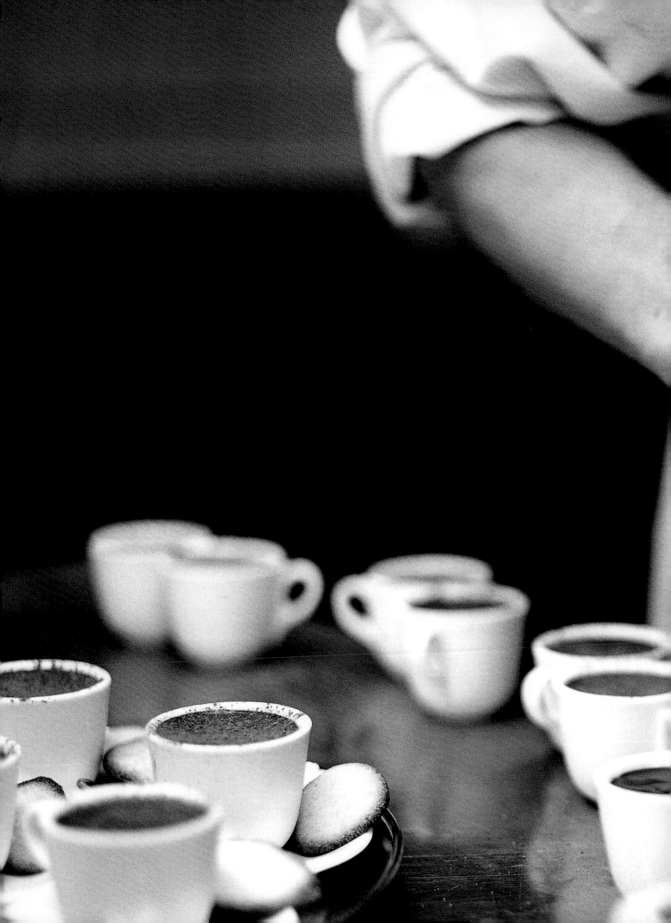

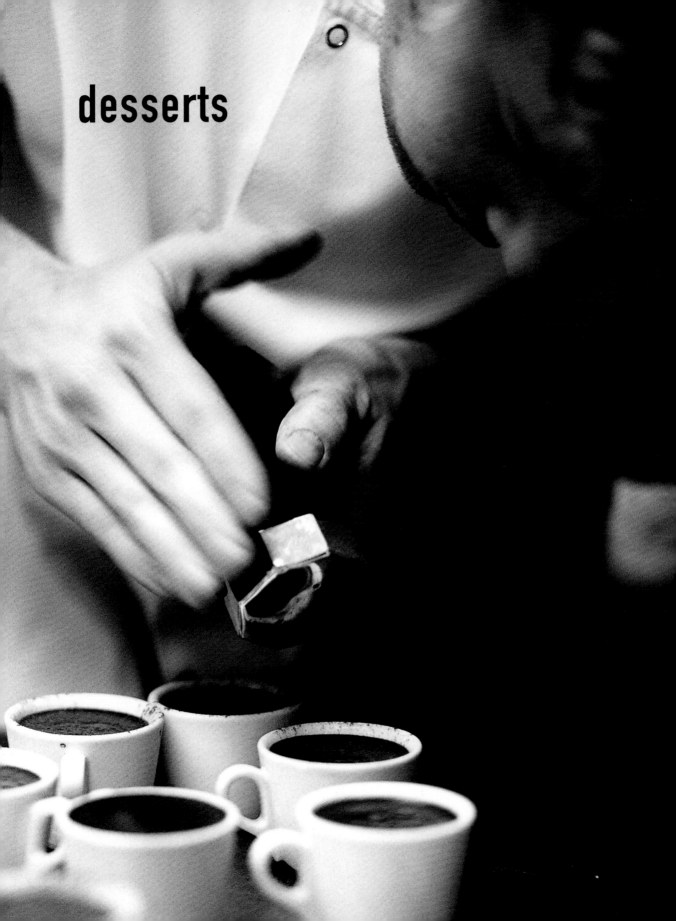

desserts

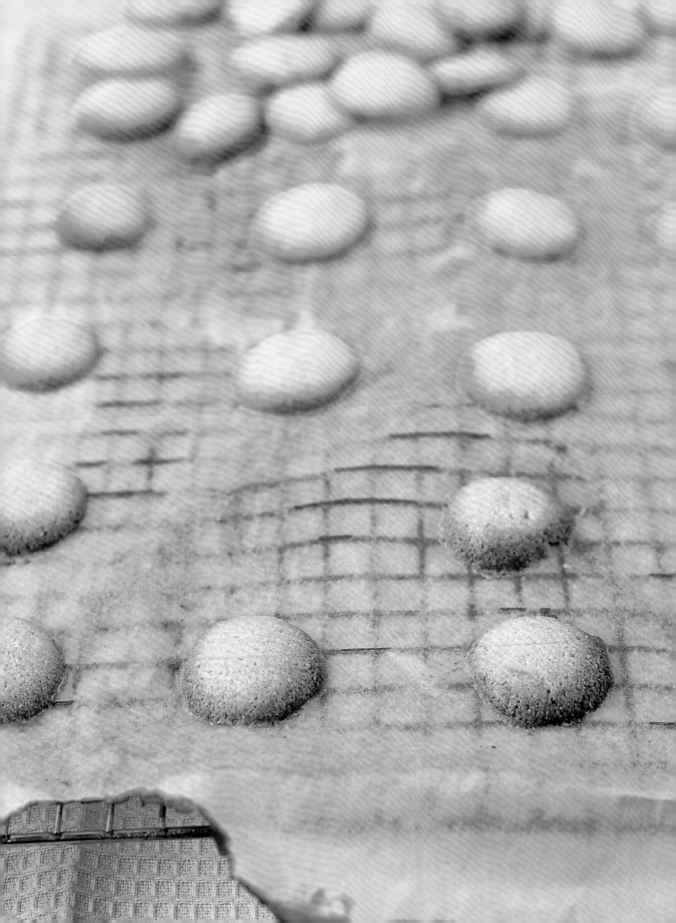

You little tiger. Naughty but nice. I can't, I can't, I can't . . . oooh, go on then. We always try to say no to dessert but, quite frankly, if you want it, have it. I'm sure I'll be quoted on this in ten years' time when I've got a workman's bum and giant lovehandles! Desserts aren't always fattening or unhealthy, but if you feel guilty after eating them then walk up the stairs instead of taking the lift, that's my philosophy. This is a small collection of tasty and very simple desserts – not technical or massively precise, which is the kind of vibe I think most people like at home.

orange & polenta biscuits

Simple and slightly unusual cookie type biscuits, with the polenta giving a fantastic crunch. Great with ice-cream, chocolatey things or a cup of coffee.

makes 25
170g unsalted butter
170g sugar
250g polenta
100g plain flour
zest of 2–3 oranges, finely chopped
2 large eggs

Rub the butter, sugar, polenta and flour together. Use a speed-peeler to peel the orange zest, then finely chop and add to the mixture with the egg. Cover and put in the fridge for 1 hour, or until slightly firm. Preheat the oven to 190°C/375°F/gas 5. Place a large square of greaseproof paper on a baking tray and spoon small teaspoons of the mixture in lines 5cm apart. Bake in the oven for 5 to 6 minutes, or until the outside edges of your biscuits are lightly golden. Remove from the oven and allow to cool for 15 minutes before eating.

CALORIES	FAT	SAT FAT	PROTEIN	CARBS	SUGAR	SALT	FIBRE
133kcal	6.2g	3.8g	1.7g	18.2g	7.3g	0g	0.4g

chocolate pots

The beauty of this dessert is that it is so smooth, silky and rich. However, if you want to lighten the texture to make it into more of a mousse, then follow the recipe here but fold in 2 stiffly whipped egg whites before pouring into the pots. Small servings are the key – I generally use espresso cups as they're the ideal size. Chocolate pots are brilliant for dinner parties as you can make them up the day before and stick them in the fridge. Ideal served with the orange & polenta biscuits on page 241.

serves 6
300ml single cream
200g quality dark chocolate (70%)
2 large egg yolks
3 tablespoons brandy, the best you can get
20g unsalted butter

In a thick-bottomed pan, heat the cream until nearly boiling. Remove and set aside for 1 minute before snapping in the chocolate. Stir in until melted and smooth. Beat in the egg yolks and brandy and stir until smooth. Allow to cool slightly before stirring in the butter until the mixture is smooth. Pour into small individual serving pots.

PS Sometimes if you add the butter when the chocolate isn't cool enough it will make the chocolate look as if it has split. To rectify this, allow the mixture to cool a little longer before whisking in a little cold milk until smooth again.

desserts

CALORIES	FAT	SAT FAT	PROTEIN	CARBS	SUGAR	SALT	FIBRE
355kcal	28.7g	16.9g	5.9g	12.4g	10.7g	0.1g	3.9g

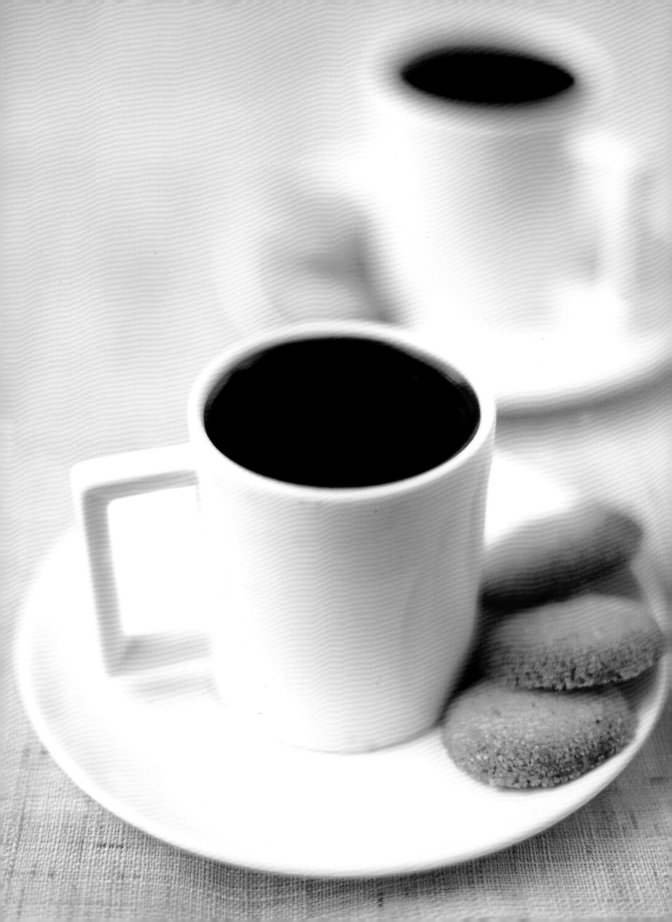

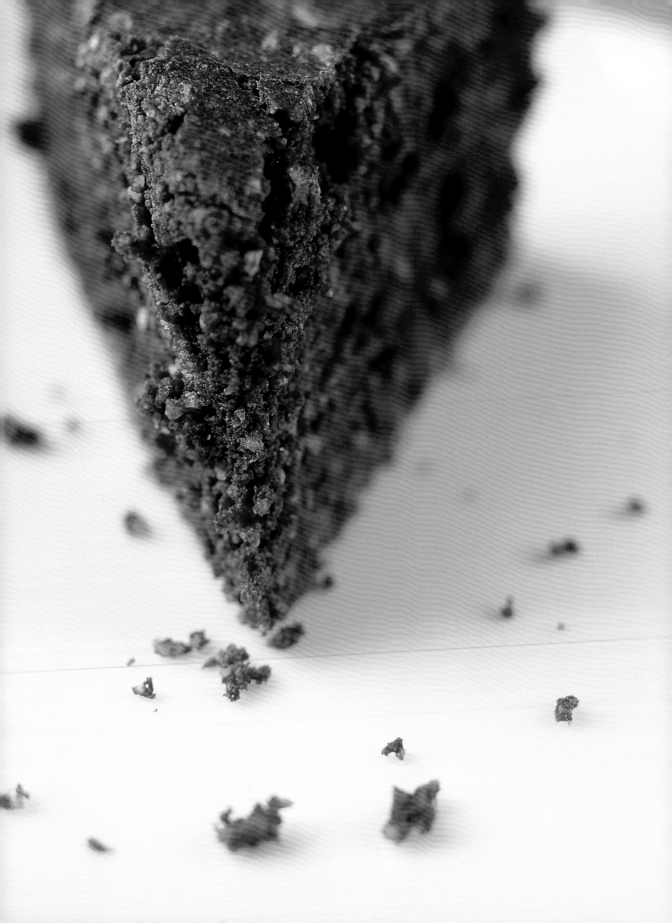

two-nuts chocolate torte

This is the best chocolate nut thang around. The day after you should try crumbling it over some ice cream with a little espresso poured over the top. I always bake this torte in a cheesecake or spring-form tin, or I make small ones baked in those trays you can use for mince pies, but you can use any well-greased and floured cake tin.

serves 12
250g unsalted butter, plus extra for greasing
plain flour, for dusting
150g blanched almonds
150g shelled walnuts
300g quality dark chocolate (70%)
1 heaped teaspoon quality cocoa powder
100g caster sugar
6 large eggs, separated

Preheat the oven to 190°C/375°F/gas 5. Line the bottom of a 20 or 25cm tin with a piece of greaseproof paper before buttering the bottom and sides then dusting with flour. Place the nuts in a food processor and whiz until finely ground, then add the chocolate and cocoa and whiz for 30 seconds to break up the chocolate. Put to one side in a separate bowl. Add the butter and sugar to the food processor and beat until pale and fluffy. At this point add the egg yolks one at a time, then mix together with the chocolate and nuts.

In another bowl beat the egg whites with a pinch of sea salt until they form stiff peaks. Gently fold the egg whites into the chocolate, butter and nut mix. Pour all the mixture into the tin. Bake in the oven for 1 hour, or until an inserted knife comes out reasonably clean. Serve with whipped cream, ice cream, crème fraîche or yoghurt.

CALORIES	FAT	SAT FAT	PROTEIN	CARBS	SUGAR	SALT	FIBRE
535kcal	46.4g	19.6g	10.4g	18.6g	17g	0.3g	3g

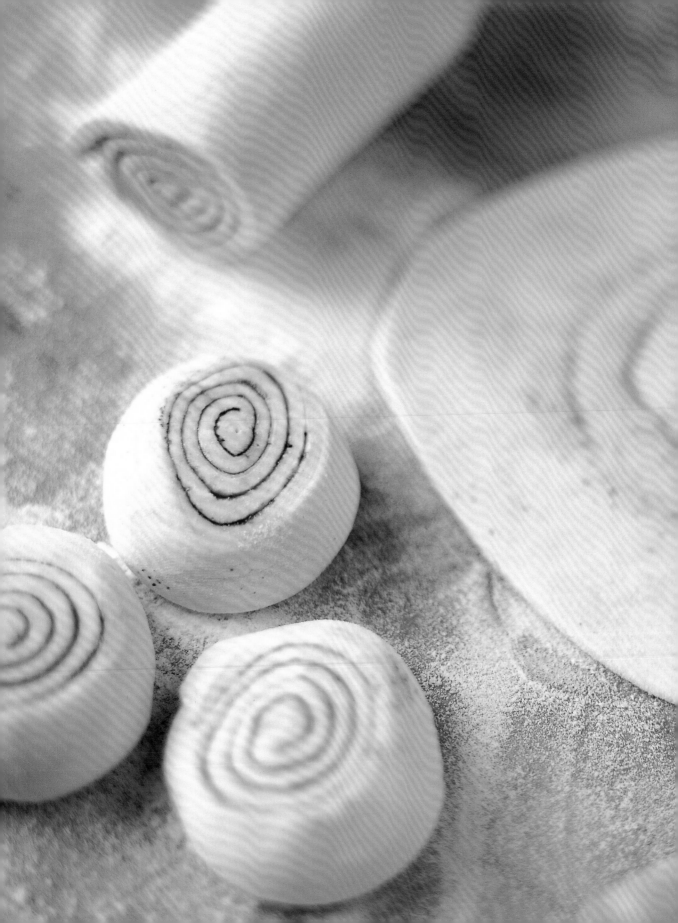

a kinda Portuguese custard pie

After eating some fantastic Portuguese cream tarts I was baffled by the crisp, light and almost chewy pastry. I tried to find out the secret to making the pastry but had no luck. So I have come up with a cunning plan to imitate it, which I think is fantastic. I found the filling kinda boring, so I've tweaked it to give it a bit of life. Might look like a palaver but is in fact the quickest custard pie around.

makes 20 pastry cases

pastry
plain flour, for dusting
250g puff pastry
1 large egg yolk
4 tablespoons caster sugar
1 whole nutmeg, for grating
2 pinches of ground cinnamon

Dust a clean surface with flour and roll out the pastry to a bit bigger than an A4 size sheet of paper. Brush with the egg yolk and scatter the rest of the ingredients over, being subtle with a few gratings of nutmeg and the cinnamon. Roll the pastry up tightly like a Swiss roll to make a long sausage shape. With a knife, cut across the sausage into 2.5cm pieces. Take 10 pieces aside and freeze the rest for a rainy day.

Preheat the oven to 200°C/400°F/gas 6. Turn all the pieces of pastry swirl-side up and flatten them slightly. Dust the surface and your pastry with flour, then roll each piece out into a thin circle (around the size of a teacup saucer). Even I don't have proper pastry moulds at home, so I just grease and flour the outsides of 10 glass tumblers. Then I place a circle of pastry on top of each tumbler, pleating, pinching and hugging the pastry around them. Place the tumblers on a baking tray, pastry at the top, and put in the preheated oven for around 15 minutes, or until crisp and golden.

Remove from the oven and, while still hot, take a tea towel and pat the slightly raised top of the pastry back down on to the flat bottom of the tumbler – giving you a flat base again. Allow to cool and carefully remove the pastry cases from around the tumblers. Fill the pastry cases with the custard filling (see page 248).

CALORIES	FAT	SAT FAT	PROTEIN	CARBS	SUGAR	SALT	FIBRE
383kcal	33.9g	19.3g	6g	17g	10.3g	0.3g	0.3g

makes enough to fill 10 pastry cases

custard
6 large eggs
4 dessertspoons runny honey
2 vanilla pods, scored lengthways, seeds removed
zest of 1 orange
500ml double cream

Whip up the eggs, honey and vanilla seeds and finely grate in the orange zest. (Don't waste the vanilla pods; simply pop them into a jar with some sugar to make a tasty vanilla sugar.) At the same time, in a thick-bottomed pan, heat the cream until nearly boiling. Add it immediately to the rest of the ingredients in the bowl, while whipping fast with a whisk for 30 seconds. Add the mixture back to the pan on a medium heat, stirring continuously and using a spatula to get into the edges. This is a very quick and almost aggressive method of cooking a thick egg custard – which is normally done in a bowl over simmering water or in the oven in a bain-marie, like a brûlée – so keep stirring to keep your custard smooth. When it gets as thick as thick yoghurt, spoon it into the pastry cases and allow to cool. A skin will begin to form on the top of each pie. To finish them off, make a little caramel . . .

caramel
1 big handful of caster sugar

Place the sugar and 3 tablespoons of water in a pan. Bring to the boil and gently agitate until golden brown. At this point it will be hotter than hot – don't even think about tasting it. No kids allowed. Drizzle the mixture randomly over the custard tarts – it will bubble and cool to a crisp caramel. Fantastic. Oh yeah – place the pan in the sink and half fill with water before boiling again – you'll have no grief washing it up.

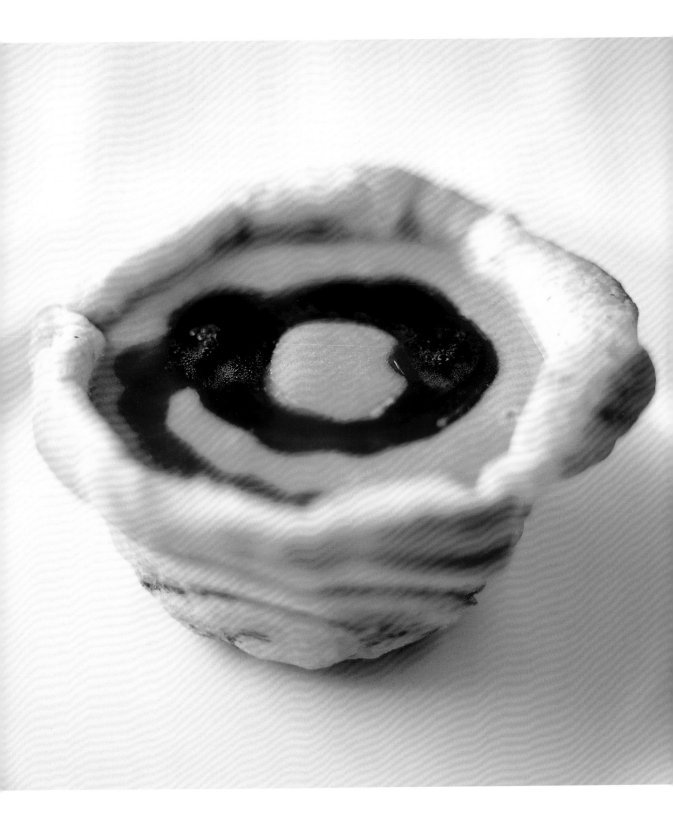

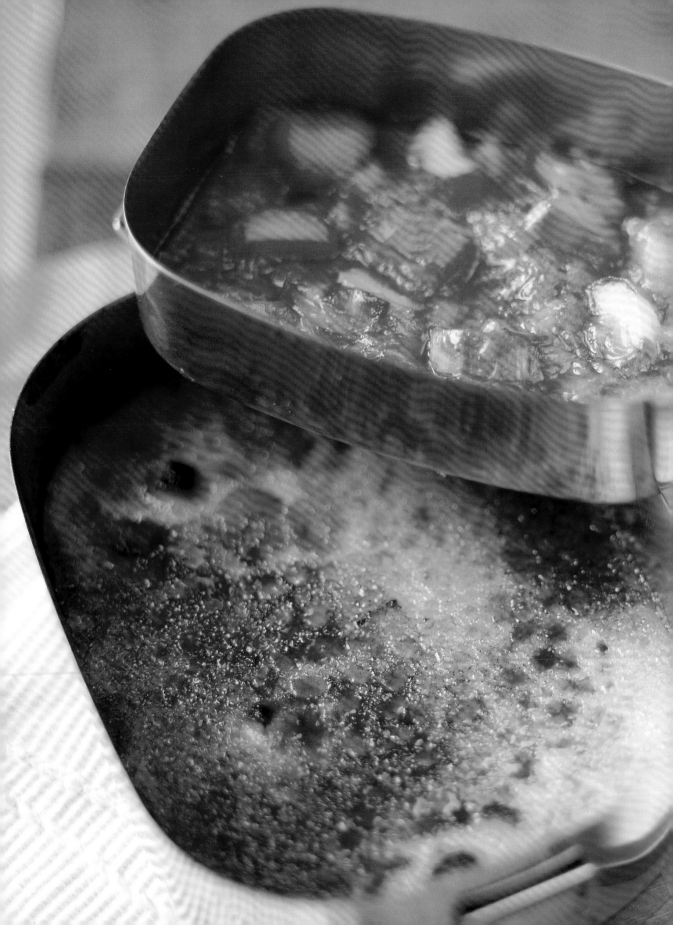

crème brûlée the way I like it

I have eaten crème brûlées all over the gaff and, at the end of the day, an egg custard is an egg custard. Some are good and some are overcooked and bad, but the most important thing is that the custard should only be 2.5cm thick, with a lovely crisp layer of thin caramel on top. So many people plonk their custard mix into a deep ramekin dish with a fat layer of hard caramel on top and that's just not right.

serves 8
300g fresh rhubarb
3 tablespoons caster sugar
2 vanilla pods, scored lengthways, seeds removed
300ml double cream
200ml full-fat milk
8 large egg yolks
80g sugar

Preheat the oven to 140°C/285°F/gas 1. Trim and roughly slice the rhubarb and place in a pan with the caster sugar and 5 tablespoons of water. Simmer until tender, divide between 8 small serving dishes which your brûlée will be cooked in, then set aside.

Place the vanilla pod and seeds in the pan with the cream and milk and slowly bring to the boil. Meanwhile, beat the yolks and the sugar together until light and fluffy. When the cream and milk are just boiling, remove the vanilla pods and add little by little to the egg mixture, whisking continuously. I like to remove any bubbles or froth from the mixture before dividing it into the serving dishes, on top of the rhubarb. Stand them in a large roasting tray filled with water halfway up the dishes, and bake for 25 minutes, or until the custard has set but is still slightly wobbly in the centre.

Allow to cool to room temperature, then place in the fridge until ready to serve. Sprinkle with sugar and caramelize under a very hot grill or using a kitchen blowtorch.

CALORIES	FAT	SAT FAT	PROTEIN	CARBS	SUGAR	SALT	FIBRE
345kcal	28.2g	15.1g	5.5g	18.5g	18.5g	0.1g	0.5g

Sheila's pudding

This is a variation of the classic Eve's pudding which uses stewed apples. I love peaches for this pudding, though many fruits can be used, such as rhubarb with almonds or plums on their own. I called it Sheila's pudding for a bit of a laugh really . . . I'm a strange boy.

serves 6

6 ripe peaches or nectarines, halved and destoned

4 heaped teaspoons demerara sugar

1 vanilla pod, scored lengthways, seeds removed

125g unsalted butter, plus extra for greasing

125g self-raising flour, plus extra for dusting

125g caster sugar

2 large eggs

Preheat the oven to 180°C/350°F/gas 4. Put the peaches into a saucepan with the demerara sugar, vanilla seeds and 4 tablespoons of water. Simmer for 5 minutes, then place in a well-greased and lightly floured ovenproof dish or bowl. Beat the butter, caster sugar and eggs together until light and fluffy. Add the flour, mix thoroughly and spread over the peaches.

Bake in the oven for 45 minutes, or until cooked through, then serve with hot custard or something cold, like vanilla ice cream or crème fraîche.

CALORIES	FAT	SAT FAT	PROTEIN	CARBS	SUGAR	SALT	FIBRE
391kcal	19.6g	11.4g	5.4g	52g	36.6g	0.3g	0.6g

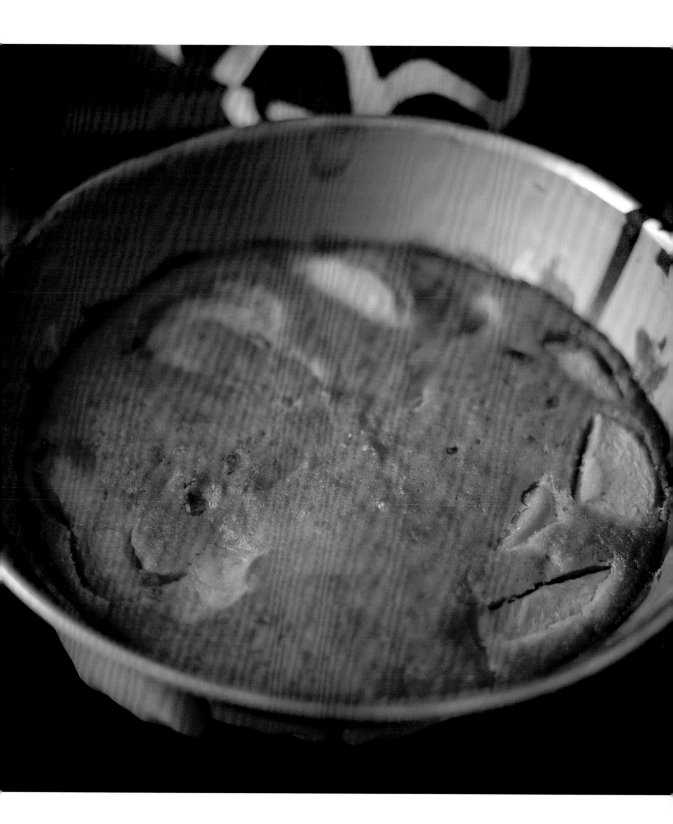

party cake

200g unsalted butter, plus extra
  for greasing
3 rounded tablespoons quality cocoa
  powder
200g caster sugar, plus extra
3 large eggs
200g self-raising flour, sifted
1 heaped teaspoon baking powder
1 handful of flaked almonds
200ml double cream

optional: sherry
1 large handful of raspberries
1 large handful of strawberries

chocolate topping
100g unsalted butter
100g quality dark chocolate (70%)
100g icing sugar
3 tablespoons milk

Preheat the oven to 180°C/350°F/gas 4. Line the bases of 2 × 20cm tins with greased greaseproof paper. Mix the cocoa powder with 4 tablespoons of boiling water. Beat the sugar and butter until fluffy, add the cocoa mixture, eggs, flour and baking powder. Mix well, then fold in the nuts. Divide the mixture between the tins. Bake for 25 minutes, or until cooked through. Allow to cool, then remove from the tins.

Melt the chocolate topping ingredients in a bowl over lightly simmering water. Stir and allow to cool. Whip the double cream to soft peaks and sweeten with a little sugar, to taste. To assemble the cake, remove the paper from both sponges. Drizzle with a little sherry (if using). Spread the cream over one sponge, then sprinkle the fruit on top. Sandwich the second sponge on top and press down. Run a knife around the edge of the cake to smooth it off and drizzle over the chocolate topping. Happy days, you've done it! Allow the chocolate topping to firm up slightly before tucking in.

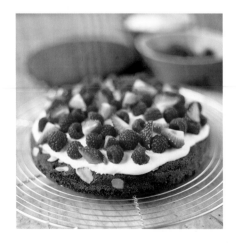 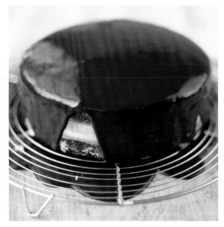

CALORIES	FAT	SAT FAT	PROTEIN	CARBS	SUGAR	SALT	FIBRE
437kcal	30.4g	17.9g	4.4g	38.9g	27.9g	0.3g	0.5g

THESE VALUES ARE BASED ON SERVES 14

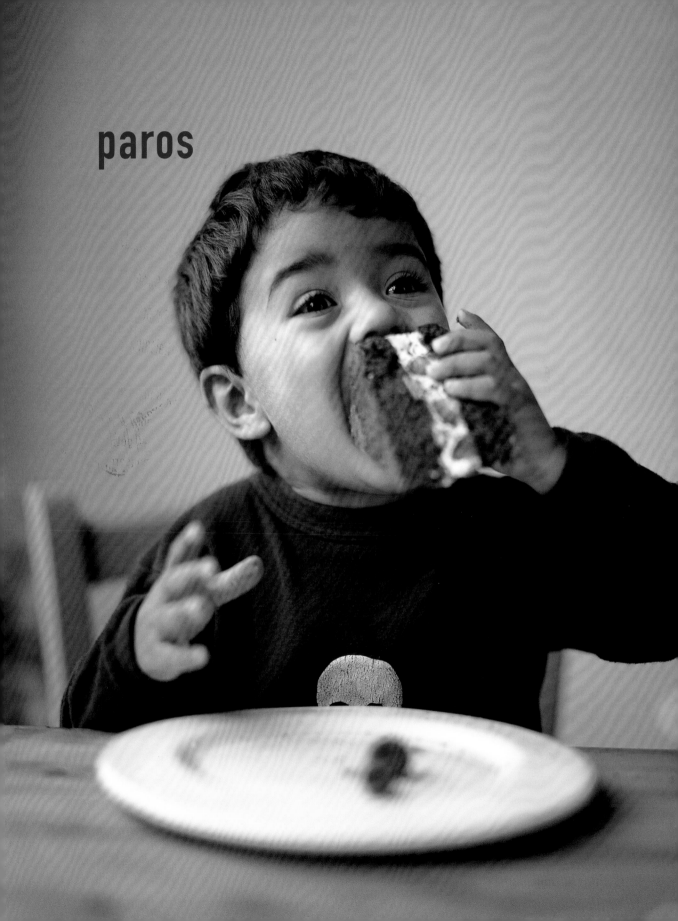

paros

strawberries marinated in balsamic vinegar

serves 4

2–3 big punnets of ripe strawberries

4 tablespoons sugar, plus extra, to taste

10 tablespoons balsamic vinegar

1 vanilla pod, scored lengthways, seeds removed

250g mascarpone cheese

4 fresh mint or basil leaves, finely sliced

When the strawberries taste pukka and are juicy like they should be, pinch off and discard the stalks, place in a bowl and sprinkle with the sugar followed by the balsamic vinegar. Stir around and allow to marinate for up to 2 hours. Mix the vanilla seeds with the mascarpone cheese and sweeten to taste with a little sugar. (Don't forget you can use the vanilla pod to flavour a small jar of sugar.) Place a big lob of mascarpone on a plate covered with a generous heap of strawberries and the tasty balsamic juice – a fine scattering of mint or basil will freshen it slightly.

   PS If you find you have any leftover strawberries and marinade, squash it all up, freeze for 2 hours 30 minutes and you've got a lovely frappé (see page 261).

CALORIES	FAT	SAT FAT	PROTEIN	CARBS	SUGAR	SALT	FIBRE
448kcal	28.9g	18.5g	4.6g	43.4g	42.8g	0.1g	7.8g

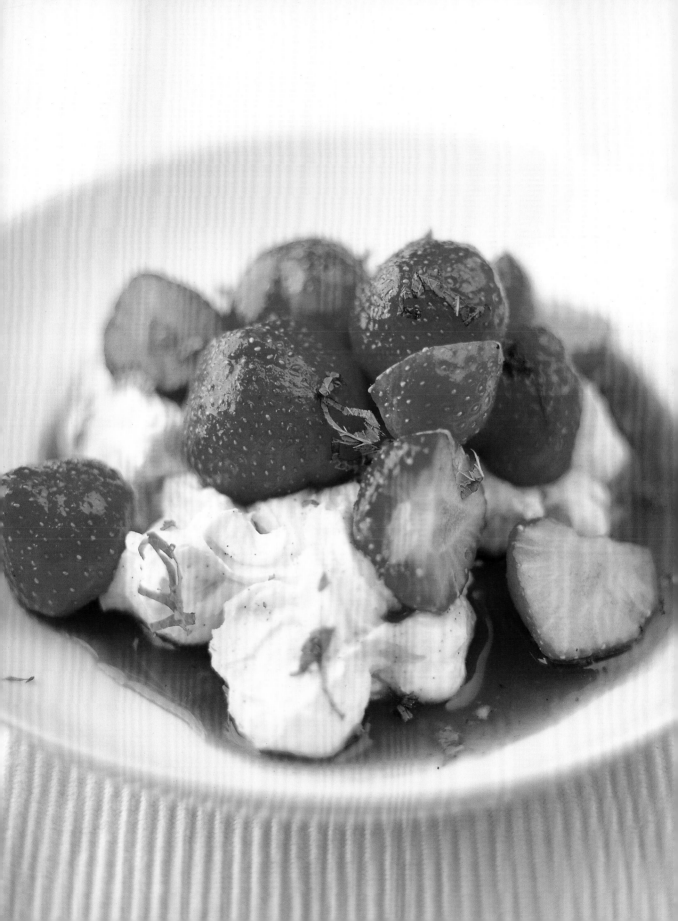

Maltesers & ice cream

serves 4
2 packets of Maltesers
1 tub of good vanilla ice cream

Bash Maltesers and sprinkle over a generous serving of vanilla ice cream.

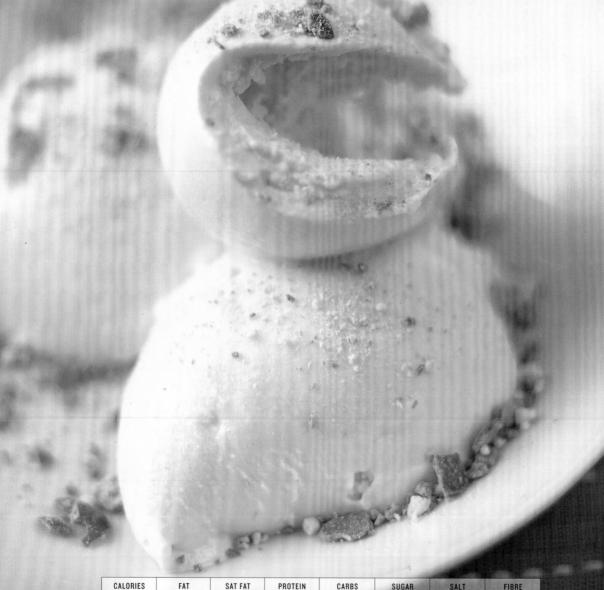

CALORIES	FAT	SAT FAT	PROTEIN	CARBS	SUGAR	SALT	FIBRE
299kcal	14.6g	9.1g	5.4g	39.2g	37.8g	0.3g	0.6g

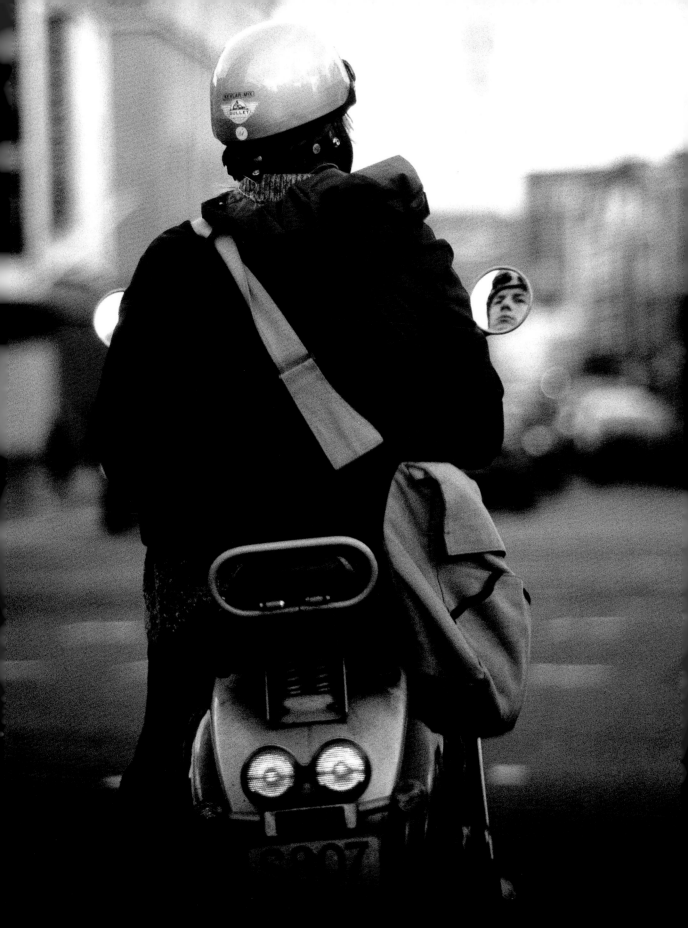

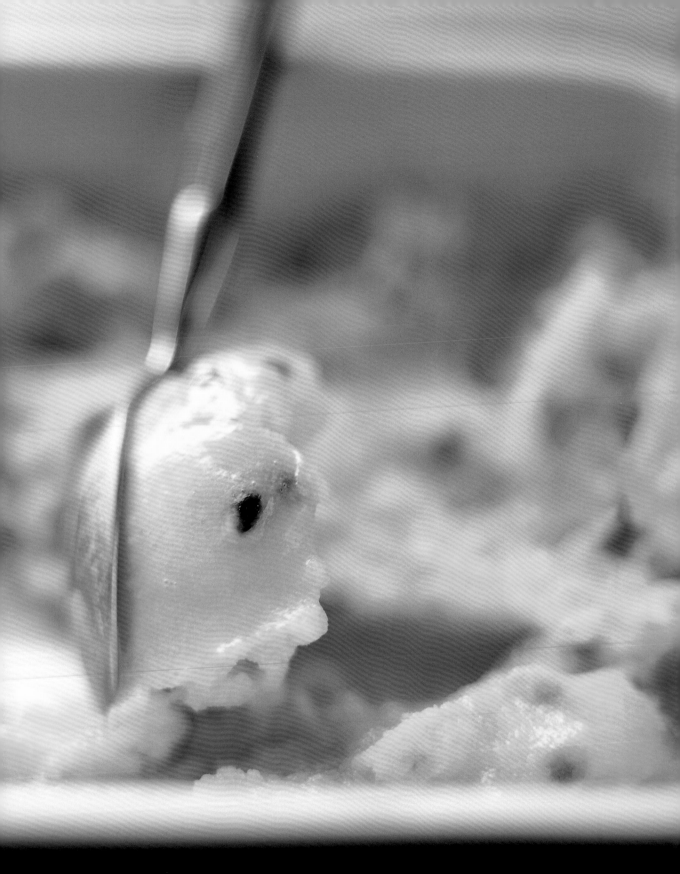

Campari & passionfruit sorbet

serves 4
200g sugar
15 passionfruit
1 wine glass of Campari

Place the sugar in a pan with 300ml of water, bring to the boil and simmer for 5 minutes. Remove from the heat and allow to cool for a while. Halve the passionfruit and scoop out the flesh, seeds and juice using a spoon. Stir this up – you can pass it through a coarse sieve to remove the seeds, but quite frankly I think that's a palaver. I like the seeds. Mix the passionfruit with the Campari and sugar syrup in a plastic tub or earthenware dish and place in the freezer. Generally, sorbet takes 2 hours to set. Try to stir it around every half an hour if you remember. Serve on its own, with some seasonal fruit, or in a cone with some vanilla ice cream.

CALORIES	FAT	SAT FAT	PROTEIN	CARBS	SUGAR	SALT	FIBRE
332kcal	0.2g	0.1g	1.5g	70.1g	70.1g	0.1g	0g

pineapple & grapefruit frappé

This recipe works with just about any fruit or combination of your choice because the principle is so basic. A frappé is basically a cross between a granita (like an icy Slush Puppy) and a smooth sorbet. As both pineapples and grapefruits can vary so much in natural sweetness, add the sugar to taste.

serves 4
2 ripe pineapples, peeled and roughly chopped
3 grapefruits, halved and juiced
sugar, to taste

Whiz the pineapple in a blender until smooth, then pass through a coarse sieve. Add the grapefruit juice and stir in sugar, to taste, remembering that the sweetness from the sugar will lessen slightly when frozen, so use a touch more than you normally would. Place in the freezer for 2 hours 30 minutes to set, stirring every 45 minutes.

CALORIES	FAT	SAT FAT	PROTEIN	CARBS	SUGAR	SALT	FIBRE
69kcal	0.3g	0g	0.7g	16.7g	16.7g	0g	1.5g

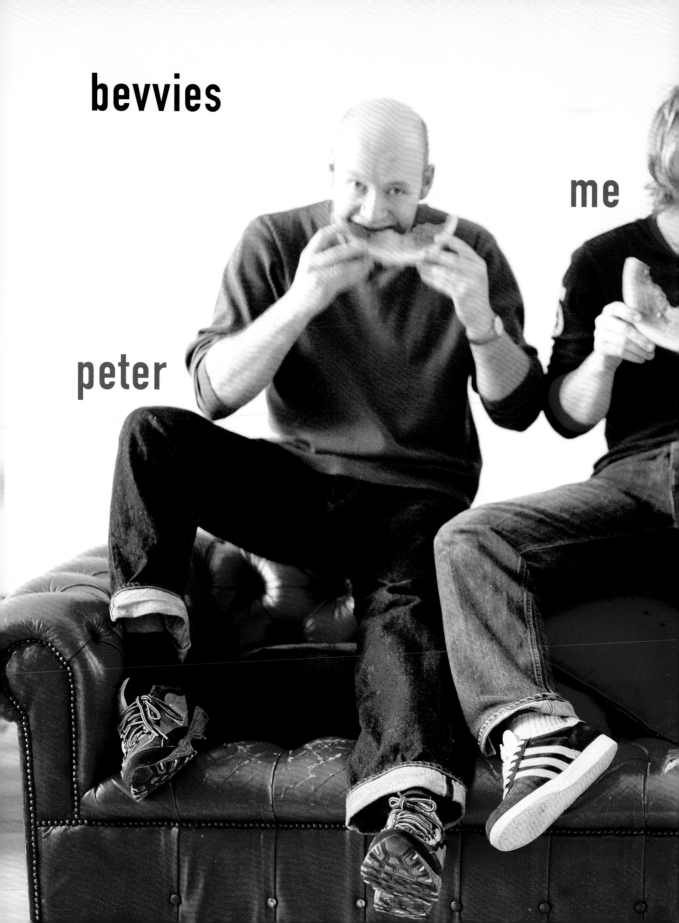

bevvies

me

peter

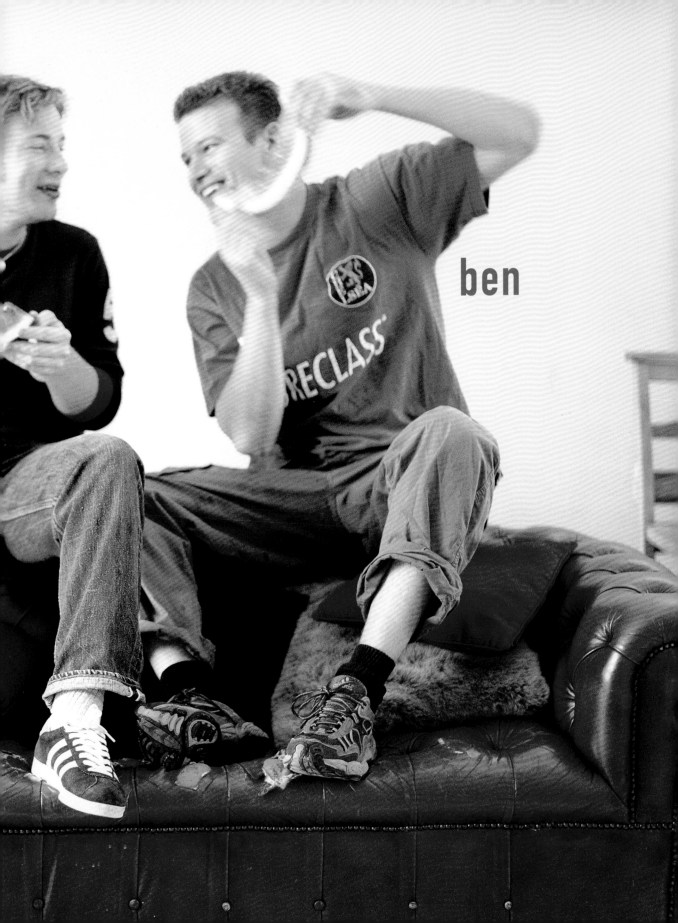

ben

When I first moved to London in 1992 all I heard with regard to cocktails and fine drinks was 'Dick Bradsell this', 'Dick Bradsell that'. His name cropped up so often I thought he was a film star. Having trained at Zanzibar in London, his precision and natural flair for mixing cocktails, and his obvious ability to evolve his drinks in new ventures, led to him setting up many great cocktail bars. With his name behind Dick's Bar at the Atlantic in Piccadilly, he also set up bars at the Soho Brasserie, the Moscow Club, the Café de Paris, Fred's Club, the Player, the Flamingo, and, most recently, Match Bar.

It wasn't until five years later that I had the pleasure of meeting him at the Player – he shook my hand and gave me one of the most memorable drinks I'd ever drunk. It sounds over the top from someone who knows nothing about cocktails, but it was bloomin' fantastic. He spoke to me for five minutes. In that time he made me realize that cocktail-making is no different from cooking. What I mean is that sometimes there are measurements and guidelines but a lot of the time it is open to innovation and natural flair. I was blown away by the way he described making drinks – his eyes lit up and his animated body language said it all to me. Passion.

I hadn't spoken to Dick again until I was thinking about having this bevvies section in my book. Personally, I thought he was the only person for the job and I knew he'd do us all proud. So we sat together and have come up with a whole range of drinks for you that can easily be made at home.

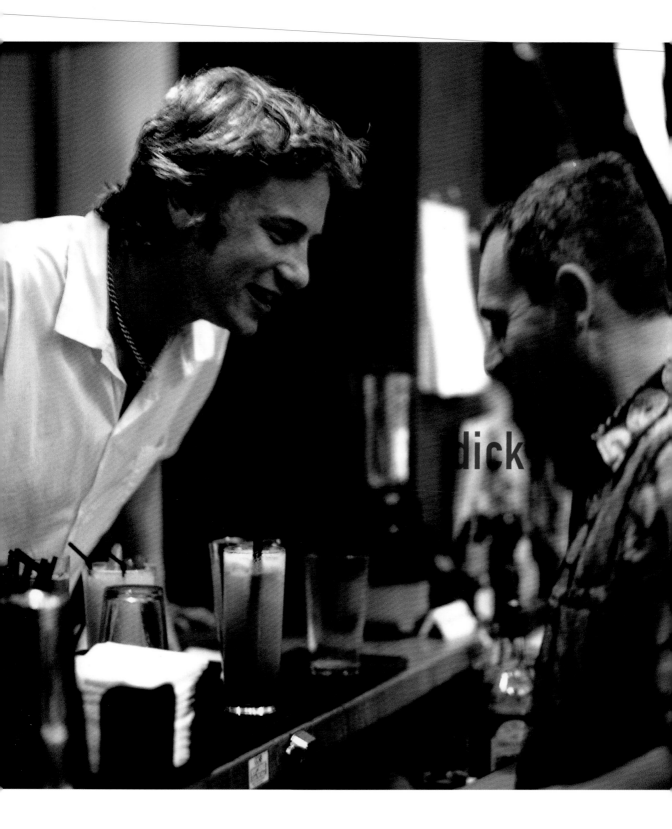

dry Martini

There are so many different ways of making this and, just for us, Dick has come up with a 'naked' Martini in the 'Franklin Style', which means it's poured straight from the freezer without being stirred over ice in the traditional way. It's named after Franklin D. Roosevelt, who preferred to have 2 olives in his.

naked

Take a frozen cocktail glass from the freezer, put a couple of drops of dry vermouth into the glass and top with freezing cold vodka or gin. Add 2 olives.

stirred

Fill a jug with ice, splash on some vermouth, stir, then discard the liquid. Your ice is now coated in vermouth. Add 75ml of gin or vodka to this and stir as many times as you like. Strain into a pre-chilled glass before garnishing with an olive or a slice of lemon.

shaken

You can shake a Martini but the result will be a cloudy drink with little bits of broken ice on top. The cocktail of choice for James Bond, of course.

CALORIES	FAT	SAT FAT	PROTEIN	CARBS	SUGAR	SALT	FIBRE
173kcal	0.4g	0.1g	0g	0.1g	0.1g	0.1g	0g

Tom Collins

The original Tom Collins employed sweet Old Tom gin, but unfortunately this is now only available in the Far East. If using London dry gin the drink is a John Collins. The vodka version is conveniently known as a Vodka Collins. Shaking a Collins and pouring it neat into a glass then adding soda water creates a Gin Fizz. And a Sling was originally the basic Collins recipe made with plain water – definitely one of the earliest of cocktails. To make the sugar syrup, mix an equal amount of sugar and boiling water together and stir until clear. Or you can buy it from any good off-licence.

Into a shaker pour 50ml of gin, 40ml of fresh lemon juice and 3 teaspoons of sugar syrup. Shake with ice and then strain over fresh ice in a tumbler. Fill to the top with soda water and stir. Garnish with a lemon slice and a cherry.

CALORIES	FAT	SAT FAT	PROTEIN	CARBS	SUGAR	SALT	FIBRE
137kcal	0g	0g	0.1g	6.9g	6.9g	0g	0g

old fashioned

This is a drink for purists. It needs a very good-quality spirit, so Dick suggests using Wild Turkey or Maker's Mark bourbon, Cockspur, Mountgay or Myers rum and any decent brandy. The idea is to take a dark spirit like brandy, bourbon or rum and bring out its natural depth of flavour; you sweeten it then give it depth by adding bitters. Perform the same ritual each time you make this and you'll get it right every time.

Take an old-fashioned glass like a whisky tumbler and pour in 4 drops of bitters and 2 teaspoons of sugar syrup (although this depends on the sweetness of your chosen spirit – brandy needs more, rum needs less). See the Tom Collins recipe on page 266 for a note about making sugar syrup, then add 2 ice cubes and stir. Add 2 more ice cubes, 25ml of your preferred spirit and stir. Then 2 more ice cubes and a further 25ml of your spirit. Stir. Then more ice and stir again. The 50ml of alcohol should now fill your glass as the ice has diluted it. Garnish with a twist of orange or lemon – lemon being particularly good with rum.

CALORIES	FAT	SAT FAT	PROTEIN	CARBS	SUGAR	SALT	FIBRE
127kcal	0g	0g	0g	4.2g	4.2g	0g	0g

Bellini

This is the famous drink from Harry's Bar in Venice, where they have a monopoly on the best peaches in the world. Over there they use the local Italian sparkling wine called prosecco. The drink tastes far better when you use this fizz, so try to get hold of some. Rather than being served in a champagne glass, the original was served in a small tumbler, but you can use either.

Use fresh peach purée if you wish. Alternatively, take a peach, blanch it in hot water to remove the skin, stone it, then blend it with a little dash of prosecco. Fill one third of your glass with the peach purée and top carefully with prosecco as it will fizz up manically. Stir as you are pouring, to fill the glass.

The junior version of this is a Virgin Bellini, where you replace the prosecco with soda. Often a dash of sugar helps.

CALORIES	FAT	SAT FAT	PROTEIN	CARBS	SUGAR	SALT	FIBRE
118kcal	0.1g	0g	1.1g	7.1g	7.1g	0g	1.1g

caipirinha

This is a traditional Brazilian drink made with the local spirit, cachaça, and the local citrus fruit, limón (little green limes with seeds). There are many different ways of making this drink – this version is the way Dick was taught to make it by an eccentric Brazilian gentleman. To replicate the flavour of hard-to-find cachaça, use almost 2 shots (50ml) of light rum and a splash of tequila.

You will need to crush some ice first. You can do this by placing it in a bag, covering it with a tea towel and bashing it with a rolling pin, as you would if you were making a crumble base out of biscuits. Take a lime, chop the ends off it and cut it into about 16 small pieces. Put in a glass tumbler, coat with about 2 teaspoons of sugar syrup (see page 266) and crush the limes to release their oils into the sugar. People often use brown sugar or white sugar in the belief that this accelerates the releasing of the oils, so experiment. You can use the rolling pin to do this, but be careful, as you're using pressure in a glass. Fill the glass with crushed ice and add 50ml of cachaça. Stir and drink!

CALORIES	FAT	SAT FAT	PROTEIN	CARBS	SUGAR	SALT	FIBRE
129kcal	0g	0g	0.1g	4.5g	4.5g	0g	0g

daiquiri natural

This drink must be made to the exact recipe measurements, as you are playing with the sourness of lime set against the sweetness of rum and if you don't get it exact the resulting imbalance in the flavour will be very obvious. The ratio is 8 parts rum to 2 parts lime and will only work with the correct rum, although other rums will have to do if you cannot find Havana Club.

For one drink, pour 50ml of Havana Club rum, 12.5ml of freshly squeezed lime juice and 1 teaspoon of sugar syrup (see page 266) into a shaker. Add lightly cracked ice cubes and shake thoroughly until the shaker becomes frosted, then strain through a mesh, such as a tea strainer, into a pre-chilled cocktail glass.

CALORIES	FAT	SAT FAT	PROTEIN	CARBS	SUGAR	SALT	FIBRE
120kcal	0g	0g	0.1g	2.3g	2.3g	0g	0g

mojito

This is Dick's favourite summer drink for when he's relaxing in his hammock. You can make this with vodka or tequila, or even cachaça if you want, but for the true Cuban feel you do need Cuban rum. Place 3 to 5 small mint leaves in a glass. Coat with 2 to 3 teaspoons of sugar syrup (see page 266) and crush to release the mint oil. Add the juice of 1 fresh lime and 50ml of Havana Club rum. Fill the glass with crushed or cracked ice. You can add a little soda if you wish. Stir thoroughly before drinking.

CALORIES	FAT	SAT FAT	PROTEIN	CARBS	SUGAR	SALT	FIBRE
129kcal	0g	0g	0.1g	4.6g	4.6g	0g	0g

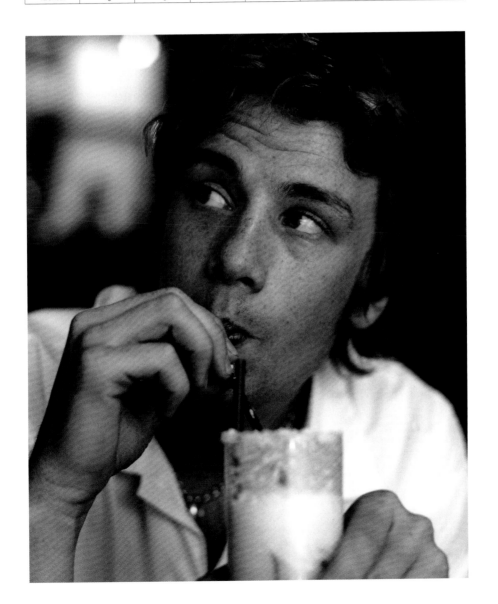

watermelon vodka

This is a really funny thing that I saw an American friend of mine make. Great for a barbie or party. Wish I'd known about this when I was going to school parties – I could have walked in with my watermelon and got all my mates completely sloshed! Needs to be started three days before you plan to eat it and is best kept in the fridge until ready to serve.

serves 12

1 large, ripe watermelon – give it a smell and
    a slap to check for ripeness
1 bottle of best vodka (or even champagne)

Simply cut a hole in the top of the melon, wide and deep enough to insert a funnel. Make sure the funnel fits quite tightly or the liquid will spill out. If that happens cut a larger hole. Pour some of your chosen alcohol into the melon through the funnel, leave to sit for a day and pour in some more. The flesh will absorb the liquid, so pour in some more the next day – basically until it becomes saturated. When ready to serve, slice up into nice big pieces and get all your mates plastered on it!

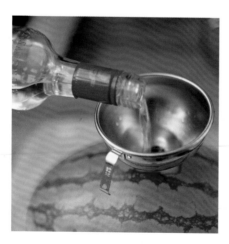
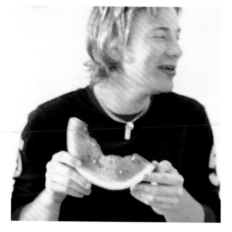

CALORIES	FAT	SAT FAT	PROTEIN	CARBS	SUGAR	SALT	FIBRE
150kcal	0.2g	0g	0.3g	4.5g	4.5g	0g	0.1g

frothy Malteser milk

serves 2
1 packet of Maltesers
250ml cold milk

In a blender or food processor, whiz up the
Maltesers to a powder and add the milk until frothy.

CALORIES	FAT	SAT FAT	PROTEIN	CARBS	SUGAR	SALT	FIBRE
146kcal	6.4g	4g	5.8g	17.5g	16.1g	0.2g	0.3g

smoothies

I love smoothies, because you can make them with anything you like. Here's a basic smoothie recipe which you can flavour with 2 to 3 handfuls of any chosen fruit, or using one of the three fantastic combinations given below.

for 2 people
1 ripe banana
2–3 large handfuls of your chosen fruit
250ml semi-skimmed milk

Place the banana and your chosen fruit in a blender and whiz for 30 seconds. Add 2 handfuls of ice and the milk. Place the lid back on tightly and pulse the blender a couple of times on and off to break up the larger pieces of ice, before whizzing to a semi-slushy milkshake consistency.

    If you haven't got a blender, place the ice in a clean tea towel and bash the hell out of it with a rolling pin, before stirring in the mushed fruit and milk.

blackberry & pineapple smoothie

2 handfuls of blackberries
1 handful of fresh pineapple, peeled and chopped

CALORIES	FAT	SAT FAT	PROTEIN	CARBS	SUGAR	SALT	FIBRE
124kcal	2.3g	1.4g	5.5g	22.1g	21g	0.1g	0.7g

banana & honey smoothie

1 more ripe banana
2 tablespoons runny honey, to taste
2 heaped tablespoons peanut butter

CALORIES	FAT	SAT FAT	PROTEIN	CARBS	SUGAR	SALT	FIBRE
333kcal	18.8g	5.5g	12.9g	30.4g	26.1g	0.4g	3.5g

raspberry & strawberry smoothie

1 handful of raspberries
2 handfuls of ripe strawberries

CALORIES	FAT	SAT FAT	PROTEIN	CARBS	SUGAR	SALT	FIBRE
115kcal	2.4g	1.4g	5.5g	19.4g	18.3g	0.1g	2.2g

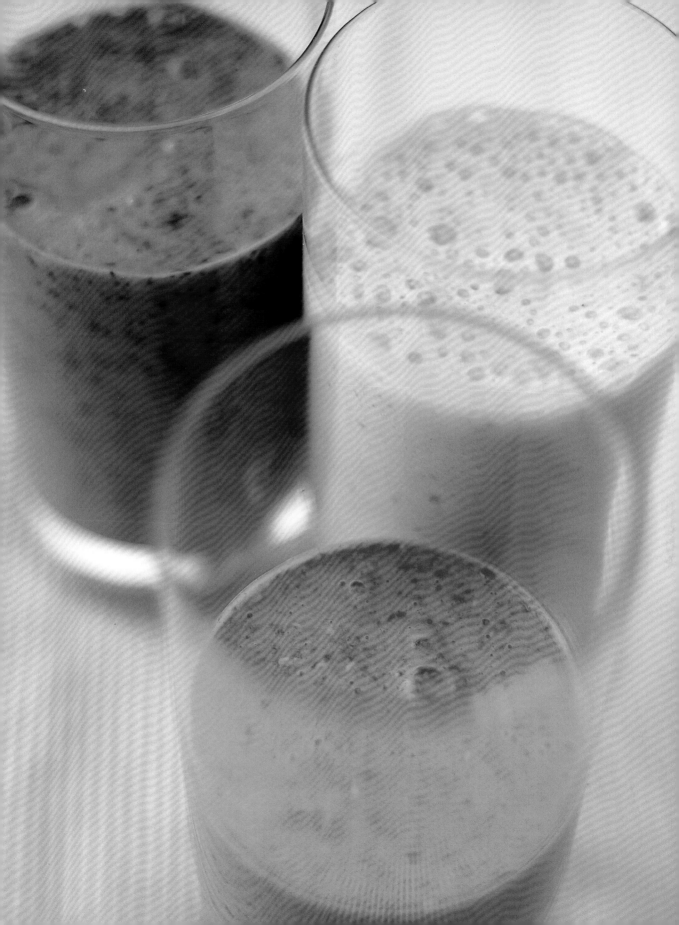

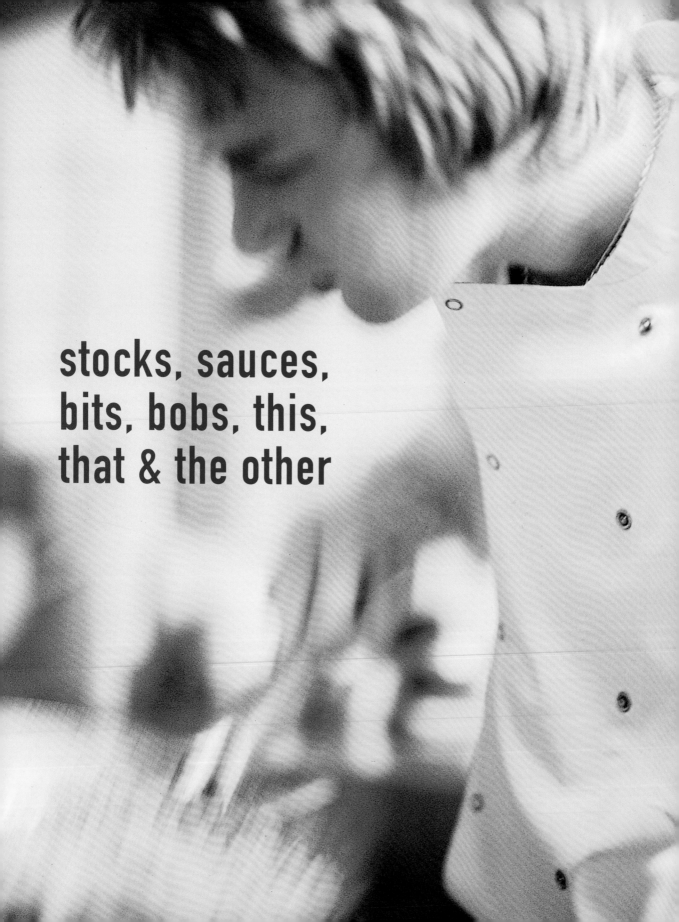

stocks, sauces,
bits, bobs, this,
that & the other

chicken stock

makes 4 litres

2kg raw chicken carcasses, chopped

½ a bulb of garlic, broken up, unpeeled

6 handfuls of fragrant root vegetables, such as celery, onions, carrots, chopped

3 fresh bay leaves

3 handfuls of mixed fresh herbs, such as rosemary, parsley, thyme

5 black peppercorns

Chuck all the ingredients into a large, deep pan with 5 litres of cold water and bring to the boil. Turn the heat down and simmer for 1 to 3 hours, skimming the surface as necessary. Pass through a sieve, and once cool you can keep it in the fridge for up to 3 days or in the freezer for up to 3 months.

CALORIES	FAT	SAT FAT	PROTEIN	CARBS	SUGAR	SALT	FIBRE
5kcal	0.4g	0.2g	0.4g	0g	0g	0g	0g

fish stock

makes 3 litres

6 handfuls of fragrant root vegetables, such as celery, fennel, onion, chopped

½ a bulb of garlic, broken up, peeled and thinly sliced

2 dried red chillies

2kg fish bones, chopped and washed thoroughly

2 tablespoons olive oil

250ml white wine

6 sprigs of fresh flat-leaf parsley

1 sprig of fresh thyme

In a large, deep pan, slowly fry the vegetables, garlic, chillies and fish bones in oil until the vegetables are tender. Pour in the white wine and cook for another 2 to 3 minutes. Add 3.5 litres of cold water and bring to the boil. Simmer for 20 minutes only, adding all the fresh herbs, and skimming the surface if necessary. Pass through a sieve and allow to cool. Fish stock can be boiled and reduced to intensify its flavour. It can be stored in the fridge for about 2 to 3 days, or you can freeze it for 1 to 2 months. A sign of a good stock is when it's tasty, clear and, when cold, sets like jelly.

CALORIES	FAT	SAT FAT	PROTEIN	CARBS	SUGAR	SALT	FIBRE
16kcal	1g	0.1g	0g	0.1g	0.1g	0g	0g

vegetable stock

Half-fill your largest deep pan with roughly chopped fragrant vegetables such as celery, fennel, carrots, onions and leeks, and add plum tomatoes and garlic, and herbs and spices such as thyme, rosemary, bay, flat-leaf parsley and chilli. If you have any dried mushrooms add them too, as they give an amazing flavour. Cover with cold water, bring to the boil, then simmer for 1 to 2 hours with a lid on. Vegetable stock will keep in the fridge for up to 1 week and in the freezer for 2 to 3 months.

garlic aïoli

serves 8
1 clove of garlic, peeled
1 large egg yolk
1 teaspoon Dijon mustard
250ml extra virgin olive oil
250ml olive oil
lemon juice, to taste

Smash up or finely chop the garlic and mix with 1 teaspoon of sea salt. Whisk the egg yolk and mustard together in a bowl, then slowly start to add the olive oil bit by bit – using two different types will give the aïoli a flavour which isn't too strong or too peppery. Once you've blended in a quarter of the oil, start to add the rest in larger amounts, then add the garlic and lemon juice, along with any optional extra flavours, such as basil, fennel tops or dill. Season to taste with salt and black pepper, adding a little extra juice to taste.

CALORIES	FAT	SAT FAT	PROTEIN	CARBS	SUGAR	SALT	FIBRE
122kcal	13.5g	2g	0.1g	0g	0g	0.1g	0g

THESE VALUES ARE BASED ON I TABLESPOON

tomato salsa

A really fantastic salsa which is brilliant served with tuna or swordfish. You can remove the skin of the tomatoes if you wish – I quite like the skin left on for this one.

serves 4–6

2 good handfuls of ripe plum tomatoes, deseeded and finely chopped

1 good handful of baby capers, soaked and drained

2 small shallots or ½ a red onion, peeled and finely chopped

½ a clove of garlic, peeled and finely chopped

1 good handful of fresh flat-leaf parsley, finely chopped

a couple of swigs of balsamic vinegar, to taste

6–8 lugs of extra virgin olive oil

dried chilli flakes, to taste

4 anchovy fillets, in oil, finely chopped

½ a cucumber, peeled, deseeded and finely diced

Mix all the ingredients together and season to taste with sea salt and black pepper.

CALORIES	FAT	SAT FAT	PROTEIN	CARBS	SUGAR	SALT	FIBRE
156kcal	14.3g	2.1g	1.9g	4.8g	4.4g	0.7g	1g

salsa verde

The secret to a good salsa verde is to chop all the ingredients very finely – fantastic with grilled meat or fish. Particularly good with sea bass (see page 156).

serves 8

2 cloves of garlic, peeled

1 small handful of baby capers

1 small handful of pickled gherkins (the ones in sweet vinegar)

6 anchovy fillets, in oil

2 large handfuls of fresh flat-leaf parsley, leaves picked

1 bunch of fresh basil, leaves picked

1 handful of fresh mint, leaves picked

1 tablespoon Dijon mustard

3 tablespoons red wine vinegar

120ml extra virgin olive oil

Finely chop the first seven ingredients and put them into a bowl. Add the mustard and red wine vinegar, then slowly stir in the oil. Balance the flavours with black pepper and, if necessary, sea salt and a little more red wine vinegar.

CALORIES	FAT	SAT FAT	PROTEIN	CARBS	SUGAR	SALT	FIBRE
137kcal	14.2g	2g	1.2g	0.9g	0.2g	0.7g	0.1g

stocks, sauces, bits, bobs, this, that & the other

minted bread sauce

serves 4
3 handfuls of fresh mint
1 handful of chopped bread
extra virgin olive oil
2 teaspoons mustard
red wine vinegar

Finely chop 3 parts mint to 1 part bread and stir in 3 tablespoons of oil to loosen. Balance the flavours by carefully seasoning with sea salt and black pepper, adding the mustard and splashing in some vinegar, to taste. The flavour improves with time.

CALORIES	FAT	SAT FAT	PROTEIN	CARBS	SUGAR	SALT	FIBRE
99kcal	9.3g	1.3g	0.9g	3.1g	0.3g	0.2g	0.1g

creamed horseradish

One of the most amazing sauces, this can turn round a simple piece of grilled or roasted beef or a roasted beetroot or carrot. Using the jarred stuff in this recipe can be delicious, but the fresh stuff is a million miles superior. If using fresh horseradish, which can be obtained from bigger supermarkets, peel and grate it.

Whether using jarred or fresh horseradish, put it into a bowl, adding crème frâiche to thin the sauce and mellow the flavour to your taste – in my case, hot. Season carefully with sea salt and black pepper and a good splash of white wine vinegar.

index

index

283

index

284

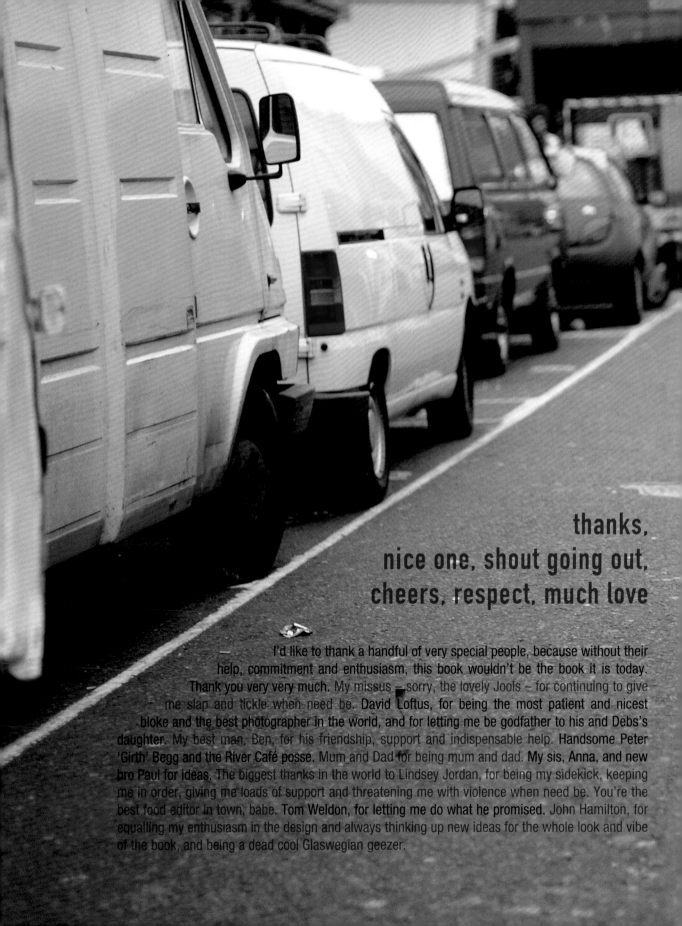

thanks,
nice one, shout going out,
cheers, respect, much love

— I'd like to thank a handful of very special people, because without their help, commitment and enthusiasm, this book wouldn't be the book it is today. Thank you very very much. My missus — sorry, the lovely Jools — for continuing to give me slap and tickle when need be. David Loftus, for being the most patient and nicest bloke and the best photographer in the world, and for letting me be godfather to his and Debs's daughter. My best man, Ben, for his friendship, support and indispensable help. Handsome Peter 'Girth' Begg and the River Café posse. Mum and Dad for being mum and dad. My sis, Anna, and new bro Paul for ideas. The biggest thanks in the world to Lindsey Jordan, for being my sidekick, keeping me in order, giving me loads of support and threatening me with violence when need be. You're the best food editor in town, babe. Tom Weldon, for letting me do what he promised. John Hamilton, for equalling my enthusiasm in the design and always thinking up new ideas for the whole look and vibe of the book, and being a dead cool Glaswegian geezer.

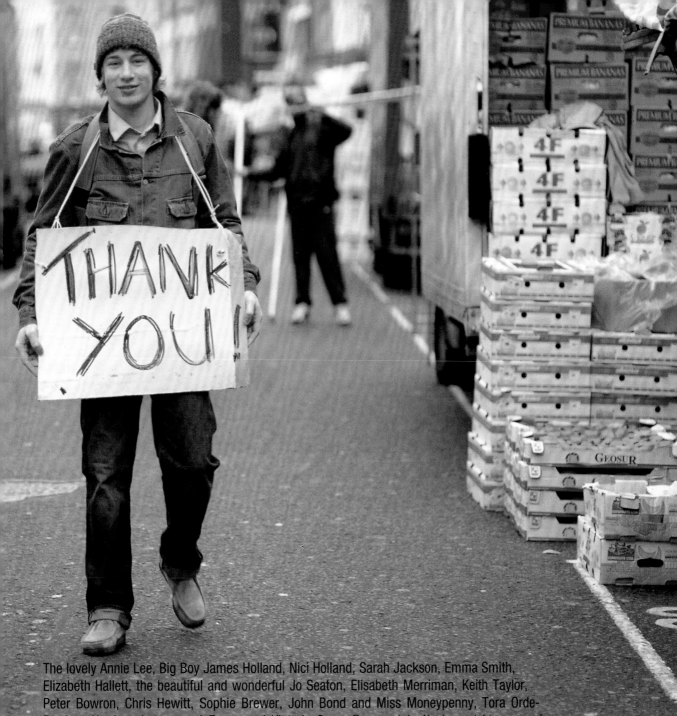

The lovely Annie Lee, Big Boy James Holland, Nici Holland, Sarah Jackson, Emma Smith, Elizabeth Hallett, the beautiful and wonderful Jo Seaton, Elisabeth Merriman, Keith Taylor, Peter Bowron, Chris Hewitt, Sophie Brewer, John Bond and Miss Moneypenny, Tora Orde-Powlett, Harrie 'what a goer' Evans and Victoria Cope. Reespect to Kevin and his mum, for Saturday soup inspiration. The team from Optomen Television: the darling Pat Llewellyn, King Kong Balls (sorry, Paul Ratcliffe), Martha, Corinne, Jessica, Richard, Jo, Luke, Mike, Bridget, Rupert, Simon, Patrick, Gabrielle, Ginny and Kate. Thanks for all your hard work and commitment. My agent, Borra Garson, and her sidekick, Michelle. Last but not least, to Gennaro Contaldo, my best buddy, my mentor and my main man. Thanks for everything. You are a handsome bastard! And thanks to my great suppliers: gorgeous Patricia at La Fromagerie, Rushton at George Allans Vegetables, Barry the Boy at Portobello Road Market and George who runs a great fish shop on Golborne Road.

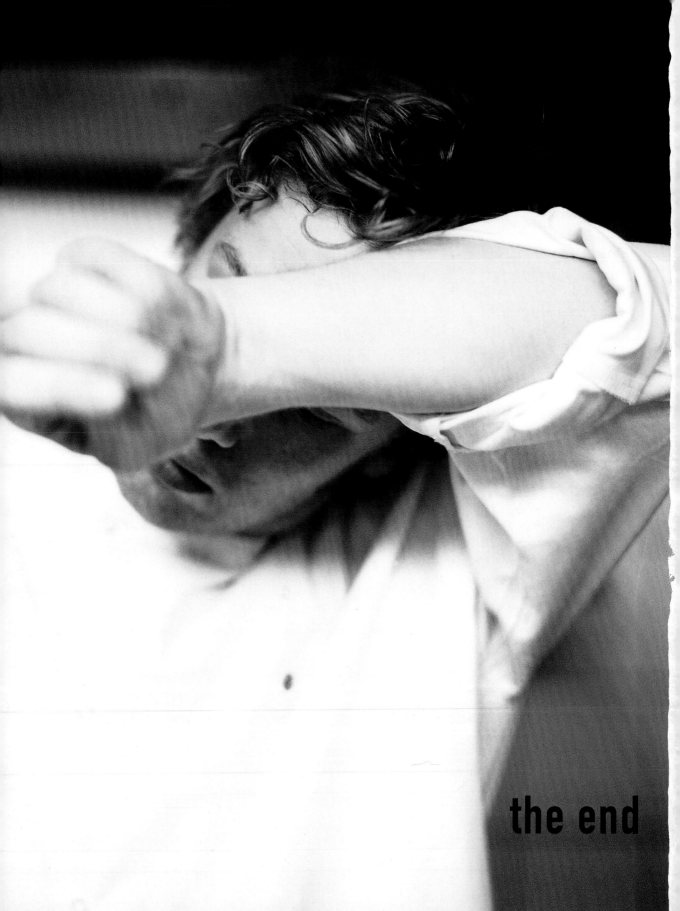

the end